MW01356072

ĪŚĀVĀSYA UPANISHAD

ĪŚĀVĀSYA UPANISHAD

COMMENTED BY

Prabhuji

Īśāvāsya Upanishad
commented by Prabhuji

First Edition

Printed in Round Top, NY, United States of America

Published by Prabhuji Mission
Website: prabhuji.net
Avadhutashram
PO Box 900
Cairo, NY, 12413
USA

Painting on the cover by Prabhuji:
"That following morning"
Acrylic on canvas, New York
Canvas Size: 48"x48"

ISBN-13: 978-1-945894-39-8
Library of Congress Control Number: 2022903775

Contents

Preface 9
Introduction 13
Invocation 17
Mantra 1 47
Mantra 2 61
Mantra 3 105
Mantra 4 125
Mantra 5 135
Mantra 6 153
Mantra 7 169
Mantra 8 179
Mantra 9 197
Mantra 10 209
Mantra 11 219
Mantra 12 231
Mantra 13 247
Mantra 14 259
Mantra 15 277
Mantra 16 297
Mantra 17 323
Mantra 18 347

ॐ अज्ञानतिमिरान्धस्य ज्ञानाञ्जनशलाकया ।
चक्षुरुन्मीलितं येन तस्मै श्रीगुरवे नमः ॥

oṁ ajñāna-timirāndhasya
jñānāñjana-śalākayā
cakṣur unmīlitaṁ yena
tasmai śrī-gurave namaḥ

Salutations unto that holy Guru who, applying the ointment (medicine) of (spiritual) knowledge, removes the darkness of ignorance of the blinded (unenlightened) and opens their eyes.

This book is dedicated, with deep gratitude and eternal respect, to the holy lotus feet of my beloved masters His Divine Grace Avadhūta Śrī Brahmānanda Bābājī Mahārāja (Guru Mahārāja) and His Divine Grace Avadhūta Śrī Mastarāma Bābājī Mahārāja (Bhagwan).

Preface

The story of my life is nothing more than a long journey, from what I believed myself to be to what I truly am. It is an authentic inner and outer pilgrimage. It is a tale of transcending what is personal and universal, partial and total, illusory and real, apparent and true. My life is a flight beyond what is temporary and eternal, darkness and light, humanity and divinity. This story is not public but profoundly private and intimate.

Only what begins, ends; only what starts, finishes. One who lives in the present is neither born nor dies, because what has no beginning has no end.

I am a disciple of a seer, an enlightened being, and somebody who is nobody. I was initiated in my spiritual childhood by the moonlight. A seagull who loved flying more than anything else in life inspired me. In love with the impossible, I crossed the universe obsessed with a star. I have walked infinite paths, following the footsteps of those who could see.

Like the ocean that longs for water, I sought my home within my own house.

I am a simple intermediary who shares his experience

with others. I am not a guide, coach, teacher, instructor, educator, psychologist, enlightener, pedagogue, evangelist, rabbi, *posek halacha*, healer, therapist, satsangist, psychic, leader, medium, savior, or guru. I am only a traveler whom you can ask for directions. I will gladly show you a place where everything calms upon arrival, a place beyond the sun and the stars, beyond your desires and longings, beyond time and space, beyond concepts and conclusions, and beyond everything that you believe you are or imagine that you will be.

I am just a whim or perhaps a joke from the sky and the only mistake of my beloved spiritual master.

Aware of the abyss that separates revelation and our works, we live in a frustrated attempt to faithfully express the mystery of the spirit.

I paint sighs, hopes, silences, aspirations, and melancholies, inner landscapes, and sunsets of the soul.

I am a painter of the indescribable, inexpressible, and indefinable of our depths. Or maybe I just write colors and paint words.

Since childhood, little windows of paper captivated my attention; through them, I visited places, met people, and made friends. Those tiny *maṇḍalas* were my true elementary school, high school, and college. Like skilled teachers, these *yantras* have guided me through contemplation, attention, concentration, observation, and meditation.

Like a physician studies the human body, or a lawyer studies laws, I have dedicated my entire life to the study of myself. I can say with certainty that I know what resides and lives in this heart.

It is not my intention to convince anyone of anything. I do not offer theology or philosophy, nor do I preach or teach, I simply think out loud. The echo of these words may lead you to the infinite space of peace, silence, love, existence, consciousness, and absolute bliss.

Do not search for me. Search for yourself. You do not need me or anyone else, because the only thing that really matters is you. What you yearn for lies within you, as what you are, here and now.

I am not a merchant of rehashed information, nor do I intend to do business with my spirituality. I do not teach beliefs or philosophies. I only speak about what I see and just share what I know.

Avoid fame, for true glory is not based on public opinion but on what you really are. What matters is not what others think of you, but your own appreciation of who you are.

Choose bliss over success, life over reputation, and wisdom over information. If you succeed, you will know not only admiration but also true envy. However, jealousy is mediocrity's tribute to talent and an open acceptance of one's own inferiority.

I advise you to fly freely and never be afraid of making mistakes. Learn the art of transforming your mistakes into lessons. Never blame others for your faults: remember that taking complete responsibility for your life is a sign of maturity. When you fly, you learn that what matters is not touching the sky but the courage to spread your wings. The higher you rise, the smaller and less significant the world looks. As you walk, sooner or later you will understand that every search begins and ends in you.

Your unconditional well-wisher,
Prabhuji

Introduction

The Upanishads are literary documents that assemble the first-hand testimony of ancient Vedic seers, or *ṛṣis,* about the ultimate reality. They are intimate revelations of those who have realized the Self. This literature has priceless maps for the seekers of Truth. These works are the legacy of the ancient enlightened sages for the following generations of sincere seekers. Upanishadic literature invites us to follow the sacred footsteps of the great sages on their path to the light. The teachings offered by the Upanishads are called Vedanta, or "the culmination of the Vedas," because for many, this collection of texts is the conclusion of the Vedas. For others, however, it represents a true emancipation from them. From a religious perspective, they can be considered a conclusion, while from a mystical perspective, they are the beginning.

The verb *ṣad* means "to sit," the prefix *ni* means "below," and the particle *upa* means "close or intimate." Thus, *upaniṣad* can be translated as "teachings received at the feet of the master." They are the specific instructions received in the proximity of someone who is able to transmit the Truth. They emphasize the esoteric nature of the wisdom transmitted by the master—who takes a seat at a higher place—to a selected group of disciples seated at the master's feet. According to the Upanishadic literature, in order to access the wisdom that it has accumulated, we must approach a bone fide master, since we can only absorb these texts at the feet of someone who has directly realized the truths contained in them.

Ṣad is also translated as "destruction." Wisdom has a destructive character because it is like acid destined to eliminate illusion. The study of Upanishadic literature brings us closer to our true nature, that is, to our most intimate reality.

The Upanishads are the final part of the set of works that begins with the four collections of *saṁhitās* known as *Ṛg*, *Yajur*, *Sāma*, and *Atharva Veda*. They were collected as written documents starting around 800 BCE in India. These four literary collections comprise the Vedic revelation called *śruti*, or "what is heard." Up through the Upanishads, India's sacred literature is pure revelation; later texts are called *smṛti* or "what is remembered" and are considered part of the tradition. The Upanishads, *Vedānta Sūtra*, and Bhagavad Gita are Vedanta's canonical texts. This literary trilogy is called *prasthāna-trayī*.

This tradition mentions 108 Upanishads, although there might have been almost 150 works of varying lengths, written in prose, verse, or both. They all focus on the same topics but approach them from a different perspective. The first chapter of the *Muktikā Upanishad* (verses 30–39) enumerates the main 108 Upanishads. The *Īśāvāsya Upanishad* is first on the list, indicating its exalted position within Vedanta literature. Although the *Īśāvāsya Upanishad* is the shortest, it has the most Sanskrit commentaries. A proper understanding of it is the key to unlock the rest of the Upanishads. Although it only has 18 verses, it is written in exquisite ancient Sanskrit and is considered to be one of the most authoritative teachings of the Vedic scriptures, or *Śruti*, by some of the most important traditional and orthodox lineages within Hinduism.

We find the *Īśāvāsya Upanishad* in the last chapter, or *adhyāya*, of the *Śukla Yajur Veda Saṁhitā*, which belongs to the *Vājasaneyi* school of the *Yajur Veda*. Another name for this book is *Saṁhitopaniṣad*, because it is part of the *Saṁhitā*, which is the collection of mantras from the ritual section (*karma-kāṇḍa*) of the Veda. This text, also called *Vājasaneyi Upanishad*, is essential in the study of Hinduism in general and Vedanta in particular, since it aims to teach the essential unity of God and the universe. Many of the greatest truths that are the pillars of Vedanta come from this short and valuable text.

The name of the *Īśāvāsya Upanishad* comes from its first mantra, *Īśāvāsyam idam sarvaṁ*, which contains one of the fundamental teachings: we believe that when we die, we abandon our belongings, possessions, achievements, and loved ones, but in fact, we leave nothing behind. In a universe impregnated with divinity, everything belongs to God, even what we are. Except for God, there is nothing.

The message of this ancient text is that the indivisible Self, the absolute One without a second, is the only reality. Everything emanates from this reality, which is the reason everything remains and returns to rest in it. It is the reality that knows all experience. It is not only the essential substance of all experience, but also the space where experience takes place.

Although we are commenting on the words from the *Īśāvāsya Upanishad*, I am not teaching Hinduism. Although we are evaluating a sacred text of Vedanta, I am not preaching a religion, a belief, a dogma, or a philosophy. My teachings are just an invitation, a few words of encouragement that might inspire you to investigate and explore deep within. By *within*, I do not mean a physical direction, but moving away from objective reality. To follow these teachings, it is not necessary to have a certain belief, but only to accept our ignorance. If we are able to observe ourselves free of interpretations, we will always find the door open.

Invocation

ॐ पूर्णमदः पूर्णमिदं पूर्णात् पूर्णमुदच्यते ।
पूर्णस्य पूर्णमादाय पूर्णमेवावशिष्यते ॥
ॐ शान्तिः शान्तिः शान्तिः ॥

oṁ pūrṇam adaḥ pūrṇam idaṁ
pūrṇāt pūrṇam udacyate
pūrṇasya pūrṇam ādāya
pūrṇam evāvaśiṣyate
oṁ śāntiḥ śāntiḥ śāntiḥ

That is the Whole, this is the Whole; from that Whole, this Whole is manifested. When this Whole is extracted, that Whole is still the Whole. *Oṁ śāntiḥ, śāntiḥ, śāntiḥ.*

Commentary:

In reference to this mantra, Mahatma Gandhi (1869–1948) said: "If all the Upanishads and the rest of the scriptures were suddenly reduced to ashes and only the invocation of the *Īśāvāsya Upanishad* remained in the memory of Hindus, Hinduism would live forever."

According to the Vedantic tradition, most rituals, ceremonies, discourses, or Upanishads begin and end with a *śānti-mantra*, or "a mantra for peace." These mantras are thought to promote calm and tranquility on all levels. Such peace is indispensable for assimilating the message. They are also attributed other beneficial properties in different contexts.

At the end of this mantra, the word *śāntiḥ*, or "peace," is repeated three times, with the intention of removing the three kinds of obstacles, or *tāpa-traya*: cosmic (*ādhibhautika*), divine (*ādhidaivika*), and human (*ādhyātmika*). The idea is that these can constitute serious impediments in the learning process.

1. *Ādhibhautika* (cosmic): This obstacle refers to afflictions arising from the *pañca-bhūta*, or "the five basic elements of nature," born from the interaction of the three *guṇas*, or "modes of material nature." Also included in this category are discomforts and afflictions caused by other entities such as envious people, microorganisms, reptiles, or beasts.

2. *Ādhidaivika* (divine): This obstacle refers to suffering caused by the anger of the gods (*devās*) or powerful higher beings for ignoring the principles of religion, or due to supernatural reasons, although in the end everything is natural.
3. *Ādhyātmika* (human): This obstacle refers to physical and bodily discomforts and diseases and to various mental and psychological disorders caused by laziness, jealousy, envy, greed, anger, rage, hatred, and so on.

The sacred syllable *oṁ* is perhaps the most important mantra in Hinduism. The *Kaṭha Upanishad* explains that *Oṁ* is so desired that human beings are willing to make sacrifices to attain it:

सर्वे वेदा यत्पदमामनन्ति तपाꣳसि सर्वाणि च यद्वदन्ति ।
यदिच्छन्तो ब्रह्मचर्यं चरन्ति तत्ते पदꣳ सङ्ग्रहेण ब्रवीम्योमित्येतत् ॥

sarve vedā yat padam āmananti
tapāṁsi sarvāṇi ca yad vadanti
yad icchanto brahma-caryaṁ caranti
tat te padaṁ saṅgraheṇa bravīmy om ity etat

All the Vedas speak about this goal and to know it well, people adopt a life of study and discipline. I am going to briefly tell you about it. This is *Oṁ*.
(*Kaṭha Upanishad*, 1.2.15)

Oṁ symbolizes the Absolute, the omnipotent, omnipresent Brahman and the source of all that is manifested. The syllable *Oṁ* is also called *Oṁkāra*, *udgīta* (the one that is chanted aloud), and *praṇava* (vibrant prayer). The *Padma Purāṇa* states that the syllable *Oṁ* is the leader of all prayer, therefore, it should be uttered at the beginning of every Vedic religious service. All study, rituals, or ceremonies begin with this sacred syllable. The *Vāyu Purāṇa* devotes an entire chapter to *Oṁ*.

It is not only the most important sacred mantra in the context of *Sanātana-dharma*, but also in the Buddhist and Jain traditions. The mantra *Oṁ* also has a very important place in the Kabbalah. According to Jewish mystical wisdom, *Oṁ* is one of the 72 names of God. According to the *Taittirīya Upanishad*, the creator Brahmā meditated on the three letters of the mantra *Oṁ* and thus arose the three Vedas *Ṛg*, *Sāma*, and *Atharva* and the three words *bhūr* (earth), *bhuvaḥ* (atmosphere), and *svaḥ* (sky). In turn, the sacred syllable *Oṁ* represents the triad (*tri-mūrti*) Brahmā, Viṣṇu, and Śiva. The syllable *Oṁ* is not only considered to be a symbol, but Brahman itself. The *Praśna Upanishad* states that *Oṁkāra* is both *parā* and *aparā*, that is, it represents both the immanent and the transcendent, the manifest and the unmanifest. Accessing the Absolute requires focusing our attention, or *ekāgratā*, which is possible through *upāsanās*, or "adorations." In general, different *upāsanās* are prescribed for various purposes. The supreme *upāsanā* is considered to be the *Oṁkāra upāsanā*.

The *Oṁkāra upāsanā* is recommended by all the Upanishads. The *Chāndogya Upanishad* states that the syllable *Oṁ* should be worshipped as *udgīta*, which is the ultimate essence of all essences.

स एष रसानाꣳरसतमः परमः परार्ध्योऽष्टमो यदुद्गीतः ॥

sa eṣa rasānāṁ rasatamaḥ paramaḥ parārdhyo 'ṣṭamo yad udgīthaḥ.

This *udgīta* (*Oṁ*) is the best of all essences. It is the best of all that exists. It is the eighth, and it has the highest status.

(*Chāndogya Upanishad*, 1.1.3)

The same Upanishad (1.2.1–7) states that the gods themselves use the *Oṁkāra upāsanā* to defeat demons. Finally, it states:

स य एतदेवं विद्वानक्षरं प्रणौत्येतदेवाक्षरꣳ स्वरममृतमभयं प्रविशति तत्प्रविश्य यदमृता देवास्तदमृतो भवति ॥

sa ya etad evam vidvān akṣaraṁ praṇauty etad evākṣaraṁ svaram amṛtam abhayam praviśati tat praviśya yad amṛtā devās tad āmṛto bhavati.

Even now, anyone who knows this *Oṁ* and worships it thus can attain the fearlessness and immortality of *Oṁ*, which is imperishable (*akṣara*).

> By becoming one with *Oṁ*, one can attain immortality, just as the gods and goddesses did.
> (*Chāndogya Upanishad*, 1.4.5)

In its first mantra, the *Māṇḍūkya Upanishad* reveals great wisdom about the syllable *Oṁ* and the *Oṁkāra-upāsanā*.

> **ॐ इत्येतदक्षरमिदꣳ सर्वं । तस्योपव्याख्यानं भूतं भवद्भविष्यदिति सर्वमोङ्कार एव । यच्चान्यत्त्रिकालातीतं तदप्योङ्कार एव ॥**
>
> *oṁ ity etad akṣaram idaṁ sarvaṁ. tasyopavyakhyanaṁ bhūtam bhavad bhaviṣyad iti sarvam oṁkāra eva. yac cānyat tri-kālātītaṁ tad apy oṁkāra eva.*
>
> This whole world is the syllable *Oṁ*. Its explanation is this: the past, the present, the future, all of this is nothing but *Oṁ*. Moreover, all that transcends the three divisions of time is also only *Oṁ*.
> (*Māṇḍūkya Upanishad*, 1)

The *Taittirīya Upanishad* points out:

> **ओमिति ब्रह्म । ओमितीदꣳ सर्वम् ।**
>
> *om iti brahma. om itīdaṁ sarvam.*
>
> The sacred sound *Oṁ* is Brahman. All of this is the syllable *Oṁ*.
> (*Taittirīya Upanishad*, 1.8.1)

In the Bhagavad Gita, Kṛṣṇa declares:

महर्षीणां भृगुरहं गिरामस्म्येकमक्षरम् ।
यज्ञानां जपयज्ञोऽस्मि स्थावराणां हिमालयः ॥

maharṣīṇāṁ bhṛgur ahaṁ
girām asmy ekam akṣaram
yajñānāṁ japa-yajño 'smi
sthāvarāṇāṁ himālayaḥ

Amongst the great seers, I am Bhṛgu and amongst sounds, I am the transcendental *Oṁ*. Amongst sacrifices, I am the sacrifice of silent repetition; amongst immovable things, I am the Himalayas.
(Bhagavad Gita, 10.25)

Oṁ consists of three Sanskrit letters: *A*, *U*, and *M*, which combine to create the sound *Aum*. The *A* and *U* are vowels, and the *M* is a consonant. Together they sound like *Oṁ*. *A* and *U* together sound like *O*, and with the *M* at the end, it becomes *Oṁ*. The vowel *A* corresponds to the physical dimension. The vowel *U* refers to the mental world, which we experience in the form of thoughts, ideas, and conclusions. *M* refers to our unmanifested state. *Oṁ* represents these three states. The letter *A* symbolizes the waking state. The letter *U* symbolizes the dream state with dreams. The letter *M*, finally, refers to the state of deep sleep without dreams. As the *Māṇḍūkya Upanishad* states:

जागरितस्थानो वैश्वानरोऽकारः प्रथमा मात्रा ।

jāgarita-sthāno vaiśvānaro 'kāraḥ prathamā mātrā.

Vaiśvānara (the subject experiencing consciousness associated with gross external objects), acting in a waking state, is symbolized by the letter A.

(*Māṇḍūkya Upanishad*, 9a)

स्वप्नस्थानस्तैजस उकारो द्वितीया मात्रा ।

svapna-sthānas taijasa u-kāro dvitīyā mātrā.

Taijasa (the subject experiencing consciousness associated with subtle internal objects), which acts in a dream state, is symbolized by the letter U.

(*Māṇḍūkya Upanishad*, 10a)

सुषुप्तस्थानः प्राज्ञो मकारस्तृतीया मात्रा ।

suṣupta-sthānaḥ prājño ma-kāras tṛtīyā mātrā.

Prājñā (the undivided consciousness, free from any experience of multiplicity), which acts in a state of deep sleep, is symbolized by the letter M.

(*Māṇḍūkya Upanishad*, 11a)

अमात्रश्चतुर्थोऽव्यवहार्यः प्रपञ्चोपशमः शिवोऽद्वैत एवमोङ्कार
आत्मैव संविशत्यात्मनाऽऽत्मानं य एवं वेद ॥

amātras caturtho 'vyavahāryaḥ prapañcopaśamaḥ śivo 'dvaita evam oṁkāra ātmaiva samviśaty ātmanā ''tmānaṁ ya evaṁ veda.

The syllable *Oṁ*, beyond all parts and all sounds, is the fourth state, transcendental, void of phenomenal existence, supreme bliss, and non-dual. Thus, the syllable *Oṁ* is really the Self (*ātman*). Whoever knows this merges their being in the Self.

(*Māṇḍūkya Upanishad*, 12)

The syllable *Oṁ* is made up of the initials of the three personifications of the triad of elements. The *A* represents Agni (fire), the *U* represents Varuṇa (water), and the *M* represents Marut (wind and air).

It is possible to access the deeper meanings of the *Oṁ* mantra, beyond its linguistic aspects. For this purpose, it is essential to focus on it, not only as a word, but as a sound. Because names are words, words are composed of letters, and letters are sounds. By transcending letters, any name will reveal itself to us as a group of sounds. Different languages are just different sound emissions. Regardless of which language we speak, if we open our mouths to make a sound, we will make the sound A. If we close our mouths and make a sound, this will most certainly be M. Any other sound is between the A and the M. If we try to find a sound between the A and the M that includes the other sounds, we round our lips to make the sound *U*. Combining the three sounds, we have the word *Oṁ*. By pronouncing *Oṁ,* we have actually said everything that is possible to say. For this reason, Oṁ is considered to be a name of God.

The term *pūrṇam* literally means "complete, whole, or totality." Only infinity can be called complete; therefore, *pūrṇa* means "infinite." Infinity is both *ananta,* or "endless," and *akhaṇḍa,* or "indivisible." In the Upanishad, the Whole or Totality is the Absolute, Brahman, the only reality without a second, and the ultimate Reality that underlies the multiplicity of the changing world. With the term *pūrṇam,* the *Īśāvāsya Upanishad* refers to what other Upanishads call Brahman. As stated by the *Taittirīya Upanishad*:

> सत्यं ज्ञानमनन्तं ब्रह्म ।
>
> *satyaṁ jñānam anantaṁ brahma.*
>
> Brahman is the absolute reality, knowledge, and infinity.
>
> (*Taittirīya Upanishad*, 2.1.1)

According to the testimony of those who have accessed this reality, it is the unique essence that lies behind all things and all beings. These sages have realized the absolute reality as their own authentic nature.

In general, we use the word *that* to refer to that which is distant, far away, or beyond our immediate reach.

For whatever is near and adjacent, we use the term *this*. *Adaḥ* can be designated as the transcendent God and *idaṁ*, his immanent aspect.

In the Bhagavad Gita, Lord Kṛṣṇa refers to the physical body as a field using the term *idaṁ*:

इदं शरीरं कौन्तेय क्षेत्रमित्यभिधीयते ।
एतद्यो वेत्ति तं प्राहुः क्षेत्रज्ञ इति तद्विदः ॥

idaṁ śarīraṁ kaunteya
kṣetram ity abhidhīyate
etad yo vetti taṁ prāhuḥ
kṣetra-jña iti tad-vidaḥ

O, son of Kuntī, this body is called the field, and whoever knows it is called the knower of the field.
(Bhagavad Gita, 13.2)

Idaṁ refers to what wc commonly consider physical, material, objectifiable, or what can be observed and perceived. This is confirmed by mantra 1 of the *Īśāvāsya Upanishad*, which calls the objective platform *idaṁ*: *oṁ īśāvāsyam idaṁ sarvaṁ*. Therefore, if *idaṁ* indicates objectivity or the manifested, *adaḥ* refers to unmanifested subjectivity. As stated by the *Bṛhad-āraṇyaka Upanishad*:

द्वे वाव ब्रह्मणो रूपे मूर्तं चैवामूर्तं च मर्त्यं चामृतं च स्थितं च यच्च सच्च त्यच्च ॥

> *dve vāva brahmaṇo rūpe mūrtaṁ caivāmūrtaṁ ca martyaṁ cāmṛtaṁ ca sthitaṁ ca yac ca sac ca tyac ca.*
>
> There are two different forms of Brahman, the gross and the subtle, the mortal and the immortal, the limited and the unlimited, the definite and the indefinite.
>
> (*Bṛhad-āraṇyaka Upanishad*, 2.3.1)

Adaḥ refers to the unknowable or unmanifested, while *idaṁ* designates the immediately perceptible, our empirical or manifested reality. *Adaḥ* means "that," referring to that which is distant, remote, or inaccessible to our immediate perception. It is not an extension in meters, kilometers, or miles, but a cognitive distance. When we eliminate the notion of length, "that" becomes "this." By eliminating the distance that separates us from what is far away, we transform *adaḥ* into *idaṁ*.

To a large extent, the information that human beings possess about themselves is superficial. In general, they know their name, nationality, profession, and marital status. If someone possesses a little deeper self-knowledge, it will be something psychological, at the most. Human beings live in ignorance about their reality. It is this ignorance that is the cognitive distance between what we believe ourselves to be and what we really are. Eliminating this distance constitutes, in short, awakening to our authentic identity as unlimited Brahman.

This verse asserts that the totality is both "that" and

"this," two statements that seem to be mutually exclusive. Affirming that the totality of "that" seems to exclude the objective, leaving it out of the totality. Likewise, asserting that the totality is "this" excludes subjectivity as an integral part of the plenitude of totality. Both statements seem untenable since they describe an exclusionary totality. When read from the perspective of *adaḥ* or *idaṁ*, the text is confusing. The correct appreciation of the text is revealed only by reading it from the perspective of totality, or *pūrṇam*.

Existence seems to offer two situations: the subjective and the objective. Besides subject and object, there is no third possibility in life. Consequently, by affirming that *adaḥ* and *idaṁ* are *pūrṇam*, the Upanishad is flatly stating that only *pūrṇam* really is. The Upanishad could have simplified its statement by just stating that the totality includes everything. There was no apparent need to divide reality into "that" and "this." However, the sage preferred not to omit or ignore our dual and relative differential experience. Our ordinary experience is characterized by the difference between the observer, or subject, and the observed, or object. In such dual experience, we do not perceive ourselves as part of the observed or *idaṁ*. However, according to the message of the Upanishad, the essence of both the observer and the observed are one and the same: *pūrṇam* or limitless totality. This is the same message that Zen Buddhism gives us in the *Heart Sūtra*:

इह शारिपुत्र रूपंशून्यता शून्यतैव रूपंरूपान्न पृथक्शून्यता शून्यतया न पृथग्रूपं यद्रूपंसा शून्यता य शून्यता तद्रूपम् । एवमेव वेदना संज्ञा संस्कार विज्ञानम् ।

iha śāriputra rūpaṁ śūnyatā śūnyataiva rūpaṁ rūpān na pṛthak śūnyatā śūnyatayā na pṛthag rūpaṁ yad rūpaṁ sā śūnyatā ya śūnyatā tad rūpam. evam eva vedanā-saṁjñā saṁskāra-vijñānam.

Listen, Śāriputra, form is emptiness, and emptiness is form. Form is nothing but emptiness, emptiness is nothing but form. The same is true for feelings, perceptions, mental formations, and consciousness.

While in the Upanishad, the nature of reality is inclusive, our dual experience is exclusive. According to the Vedantic message, the subject–object relationship is inclusive, whereas our relative dual experience is one of complete differentiation between the two. By excluding the observed, human beings perceive themselves as incomplete in their ordinary experience. It is from such a partial and illusory perception that a deep sense of dissatisfaction originates.

Plenitude, or *pūrṇam*, is all-inclusive.

It is impossible to limit wholeness within a form. Any outline, whether physical, material, astral, ghostly, or spiritual, implies a boundary or limit. A silhouette that does not demarcate an inside and an outside is meaningless as a form. From our relative and partial perspective, we perceive ourselves as bounded within a limited world that is different from us. We perceive the limitation of an objective world distinct from the perceiver. The experience of a difference between subject and object conflicts with the assertion in the Upanishads that the essence of both the observer and the observed is *pūrṇam*. Diversity necessarily implies limitation. As long as we feel limited and incomplete, we will continue to strive to escape such a feeling and try to complete ourselves through different means that supposedly offer temporary satisfaction. The dissatisfaction that accompanies human beings comes from limited self-perception.

The pursuit of pleasure, enjoyment, and happiness is intimately linked to this sense of limitation. According to Vedanta, such a search is futile because we are eternally unlimited. Although our nature is limitless totality, the Upanishad accepts our dual experience of differentiation by using terms such as "that" and "this." *Adaḥ* refers to subjectivity, which appears to be different from the observed. *Idaṁ* refers to objectivity, which appears to be different from the observer and reveals differences between objects. Although it appears to be subjectivity and objectivity, *pūrṇam* includes everything. Vedanta denies the reality of dual experience, but does not discredit the experience itself. The sages of yore did not deny subject–object experience, but rather that this was absolute reality; they accepted it as relative experience.

If dual objective experience had not been accepted as *pūrṇam*, then *pūrṇam* would have been relegated to only an undifferentiated subjective experience. If so, such an experience would be pursued as an escape from dual experience, which is supposedly devoid of *pūrṇam*. But *mokṣa*, or "liberation," cannot come from an escape because such a liberation would only be a reaction to the illusion and, thus, part of it. Enlightenment is not like a glass of whiskey or a marijuana cigarette. It is impossible to reduce liberation to an experience, however beautiful it may be, because every experience is limited, relative, and temporary.

Vedanta does not reject the dual subject–object experience, but rejects the conclusion that we are something other than what is perceived. Duality is experience, but not reality. The illusion of human beings does not consist in experiencing duality, but in concluding that such experience is real.

If we dream that we study medicine, we will not receive a diploma when we wake up. If we dream that we win the lottery, there will be no change in our bank account balance when we open our eyes in the morning. During the dream, the experience was indisputably real, but upon awakening we realized that it was only a dream.

The Vedantic negation of our dualistic conclusion of reality is not based on faith, but on *śruti* as *pramāṇa*. The revealed scriptures not only have a theological and mythological value, but they are a valid means of accessing knowledge. Each means of acquiring knowledge, or *pramāṇa,* provides access to a specific piece of valid knowledge, just as each sense is a means to perceive specific information from the empirical universe. Just as the eye gives us access to color and form and the ear to sound, the revealed scriptures are the means to attain knowledge of the ultimate Reality. Upanishadic statements heard directly from the lips of a truly realized master are an effective means of attaining valid knowledge about our authenticity.

According to Aristotle, the material cause is the material used for creation, while the efficient cause is the creator. For example, in a painting, we would say that the canvas and paint are the material cause and the painter is the efficient cause. The universe raises two questions for us: what is its material cause, or *upādāna-karana*, and what is the efficient cause, or *nimitta-kāraṇa*? The Upanishads establish Brahman as the material cause of the universe.

यतो वा इमानि भूतानि जायन्ते । येन जातानि जीवन्ति ।
यत्प्रयन्त्यभिसंविशन्ति । तद्विजिज्ञासस्व । तद्ब्रह्मेति ।

yato vā imāni bhūtāni jāyante. yena jātāni jīvanti. yat prayanty abhisaṁviśanti. tad vijijñāsasva. tad brahmeti.

Seek to know that from which all beings here are born; having been born, by which they remain alive; and into which, on departing, they enter. That is Brahman.

(*Taittirīya Upanishad*, 3.1.1)

Vedanta automatically refers to Brahman as the efficient cause. However, the scriptures do not directly say it is the efficient cause. Since the existence of more than one unlimited totality is impossible, an unlimited material cause necessarily excludes the existence of a second unlimited efficient cause. The Upanishad asserts that both subjectivity and objectivity are *pūrṇam* or Brahman; therefore, both share the same efficient and material cause. As effects of the same cause, subject and object are essentially identical. If an efficient cause were needed, the God creator of the universe would be an integral part of the totality, or *pūrṇam*. The phenomenon of sleeping with dreams is a good example of an experience in which diverse effects share the same cause, both material and efficient. The dreamer is both the material and efficient cause of the dream, since both the substance of the dream and its creator come from the dreamer.

The dream is a dual experience in which a subject–object relationship is established. However, the separation in the dream is false, since the matter that all the objects and characters are made of is the very dreamer. Within the dream, you are both the observer and the observed, both the subject and the object. With some resemblance to the first part of the mantra, we would say that both the efficient and material cause are *pūrṇam* or Brahman. As with the dreamer, *pūrṇam* dilutes all apparent difference between subjectivity and objectivity. The Upanishad's affirmation that the totality is "this" and "that" eliminates the apparent subject–object difference that we experience.

***Pūrṇāt pūrṇam udacyate* or "from that Whole, this Whole is manifested."**

The first line of the mantra says *oṁ pūrṇam adaḥ pūrṇam idaṁ*: "That (*adaḥ*) is the Whole (*pūrṇam*), this (*idaṁ*) is the Whole." The second line says: *pūrṇāt* (of the totality) *pūrṇam* (the totality) *udacyate* (originates). Looking at the grammatical word order, it is clear that the Upanishad refers to a relationship of apparent cause and effect between the amorphous *pūrṇam* (*adaḥ* – mentioned first in the previous sentence) and the form-possessing *pūrṇam* (*idaṁ* – mentioned second). Thus, the translation of *pūrṇāt pūrṇam udacyate* would be "from that Whole, this Whole is manifested." This part of the mantra refers to a creation whose reality, according to Vedanta, is *mithyā*, or "illusory." It is like a mirage in the desert, where reality is not absolute; it is only empirical and phenomenal. In the same way, the non-existent serpent "this" manifests from the rope "that," which does exist.

According to our ordinary experience, the effect produces a mutation in its respective cause. The making of every piece of wood furniture affects a tree. If we buy a new house or a car, the consequence is that our bank balance will be affected. However, the statement in this mantra would seem to challenge ordinary mathematics. According to the mantra *pūrṇasya pūrṇam ādāya pūrṇam evāvaśiṣyate*, "When this Whole is extracted, that Whole remains being the Whole." The phenomenal world, immediately accessible to our senses (this), consists of a projection onto consciousness (that). Ultimate reality, like the rope, is neither reduced by the appearance of the serpent nor increased by its removal. The Absolute is not affected by the appearance and disappearance of the relative. The drama that unfolds in the film does not affect the screen in the movie theater.

In general, in any cause–effect relationship, we assume that the cause undergoes a change to produce the effect. However, although it is the cause of the entire universe, Brahman remains immutable. Its apparent mutability can be compared to the change gold undergoes when making of a piece of jewelry. Gold is extracted from a mine and melted down. The gold is not affected when it is used to make a bracelet, a pair of earrings, or a ring. Likewise, it is possible to create a universe from *pūrṇam* without affecting it.

Pūrṇāt pūrṇam udacyate, the omission of *adaḥ* and *idaṁ* clearly establishes that only *pūrṇam* really is. Just as clay does not undergo a change when used to make jars or vases, *pūrṇam* remains immutable, even though objective diversity (*idaṁ*) arises from it.

It is not easy to differentiate cause from effect. For example, it would be a mistake to say that the clay vase is an effect of the clay. The clay vase is not completely different from clay, but it is clay. The production of such a vase does not result in two distinct products, the vase and the clay. Although we see a clay vase before us, the clay has not been removed. The vase and the clay do not constitute two essentially different realities. This example helps us understand that on the empirical plane, the effect is not completely different from its material cause. If we understand that the effect is an expression of its cause, we will accept them both as one and the same. Likewise, although we perceive a diversity of names and forms through our senses, in reality, only *pūrṇam* is.

The first *śloka* of the *Catuḥ-ślokī Bhāgavatam* states:

अहमेवासमेवाग्रे नान्यद्यत्सदसत्परम् ।
पश्चादहं यदेतच्च योऽवशिष्येत सोऽस्म्यहम् ॥

aham evāsam evāgre
nānyad yat sad-asat param
paścād ahaṁ yad etac ca
yo 'vaśiṣyeta so 'smy aham

Before creation, I alone existed, there was nothing superior or different from me in the form of real (*sat*) or unreal objects (*asat*), which are illusions. Also, after [creation] began, I was all that existed. Once this [creation] ends, I will be all that remains.
(*Catuḥ-ślokī-bhāgavatam*, *Śrīmad-bhāgavatam*, 2.9.33)

***Pūrṇam evāvaśiṣyate* or "that Whole remains the Whole."**

That is to say, if we extract the objective from the subjective or adhere to it, all that remains is the totality. If we withdraw *idaṁ pūrṇam*, or objectivity, from *adaḥ pūrṇam*, or subjectivity, or adhere *idaṁ pūrṇam* to *adaḥ pūrṇam*, all that remains will be *pūrṇam*. Even if the gold is shaped into a ring or bracelet, it will not cease to be gold. Even if we melt the ring, it will still be gold.

Pūrṇam or Brahman is immutable; it is not necessary to melt the jewelry to perceive the gold. Many believe that in order to realize consciousness, the world and its diversity must evaporate. But it is not necessary to destroy the shirt to appreciate the silk it is made of. The perception of clay is not conditioned by the destruction of the pot. Similarly, it is not essential that the phenomenal world be eliminated or the dual experience disappear in order to experience *pūrṇam*. It is possible to perceive gold by only observing bracelets, chains, earrings, and rings. Gold jewelry will never be something other than gold. It is possible to enjoy the experience of observing the ocean while still seeing the waves, because the waves are the ocean. Likewise, the Upanishad uses terms like adding and subtracting to facilitate our understanding that nothing affects Brahman. By bestowing names and forms on the unlimited Brahman, nothing is added or attached to it. Nor by subtracting creation is *pūrṇam* affected at all.

What can be denied is not real. Clearly, reality does not allow negation. However, every object lacks reality because it is deniable in both time and space. Any difference in the objective dimension is illusory. The objective world does not have a real independent existence. Since it is superimposed onto Brahman, its existence depends entirely upon *pūrṇam*. Examining an object, we will see that it is only a name and a form, reducible to another substance. In turn, this substance is a name and a form, reducible to other micro-substances. Therefore, everything that can be objectified eludes an ultimate definition since it lacks a reality of its own. Objectivity consists of names and forms, in a constant process of mutation, limited by space and time whose reality is sustained by Brahman. By observing different objects, it is possible to perceive their lack of differences. They consist only of limited, reducible, and deniable names and forms, and their differences are soluble in Brahman. Because they lack true substantiality, objects are not really different from each other.

In terms of the efficient cause, I would say that creation cannot be properly understood as an act separate from the creator. Ordinary human beings create effects from their activities because they act believing they are subjects that are distinct from their activities. But an action of totality cannot be considered an activity because totality includes everything. If nothing exists outside *pūrṇam*, it includes both itself and its own actions.

If we extract a portion of something, obviously the

source will decrease proportionally to what is extracted. Following the same reasoning, we would say that if God is the origin of the universe, he should have diminished with the creation of the universe. However, we read in the Upanishad that God did not diminish after creating the universe. It is impossible to subtract anything from the unlimited totality. If it included everything, we would need a space free from totality to place what was extracted.

Within our relative understanding, we think that the effect reduces the substance of its cause. However, such a view is based on the law of cause and effect that prevails in the context of our dual reality of subject and object. According to the Upanishad, if we subtract something from the totality, the totality is not reduced. Thus, the emanation of the universe has not caused any reduction of the totality. Likewise, every action in the unlimited totality lacks an effect separate from its cause, as if nothing had ever happened. On our relative and dual dimension, what we do is not the same as what we are; our activities are modifications of our personality. But on the absolute level, there is no difference between God's existence and actions.

Activity and action, although similar, are not the same. Action does not exist separately from being. However, unlike action, activity binds and enslaves us through its reactions or effects. We can only conceive of ourselves as active if our activity is different from what we are. If our action is intrinsic to our being, we can consider ourselves inactive. Such action does not enslave or limit us because it is not something we do, but it is what we are. It is not about our activity, but about us. The law of cause and effect is only relevant on the dual plane, along with the notions of subject and object. The profound interdependence that exists in the universe does not allow for the existence of a cause separate from an effect. If we perceive the universe holistically as an organism, we cannot accept the independent functioning of one of its parts. Like a wave in the sea, we flow through our actions until they disappear, leaving room for only the ocean of consciousness. Likewise, instead of activity, only the unchanging Self remains. What is called *yoga*, or "union," is just that: the integration of being and doing. In our dual and relative reality, the experience is one of conflict and disintegration. We strive to complete our inner world through our contact with the empirical world via the senses. The existence of such an objective reality depends on our sensory perception. However, God's activity does not consist in the result of what an actor or creator does. In that sense, God's creative activity cannot be categorized as true activity. In the Bhagavad Gita, Kṛṣṇa clearly states:

चातुर्वर्ण्यं मया सृष्टं गुणकर्मविभागशः ।
तस्य कर्तारमपि मां विद्ध्यकर्तारमव्ययम् ॥

cātur-varṇyaṁ mayā sṛṣṭaṁ
guṇa-karma-vibhāgaśaḥ

tasya kartāram api māṁ
viddhy akartāram avyayam

> The four-fold caste system has been created by me according to the differentiation of qualities and actions. Though I am the author, know me as non-doer and eternal.
>
> (Bhagavad Gita, 4.13)

God and God's action are one and the same. Although he has created everything, in reality, God has never done anything. The unlimited totality manifests itself as the universe without diminishing the content of God. The theory of a creation originating in a creator is based on the idea of cause and effect. However, this law is totally irrelevant in the absence of factors such as space or time. These factors, which result from creation, are clearly subsequent to it. Consequently, it is impossible for them to affect God. If we understand that the principle of cause and effect cannot be applied to God, it is absurd to conceive of creation as an effect and God as its cause. God is *sarva-kāraṇa-kāraṇam*, or the "prime cause of all causes," without actually being the cause of anything. Although God is generally regarded as the source of the universe, in fact nothing ever happened because God never created anything. God, or the immutable totality, remains the same as before the creation that we try to attribute to him.

For many, it is difficult to understand that the universe

we perceive has never really been created. Especially because we look around and see a variety of tangible objects such as chairs, tables, trees, and people. It is possible to see and touch all these solid objects. However, if we look at a tree with a powerful microscope, the tree will no longer be a solid object but a cluster of molecules. If we use an even more powerful microscope, the molecules will disappear and we will see different particles called atoms. If we get an even more powerful microscope, we will see even smaller microparticles that are extremely different from the atoms. The tree disappears to give rise to inconceivable quantum spaces. Thus, we understand that there has never been a tree, but our vision and physical conditions have shown us something solid made of microparticles. Such a sea of particles have never been a tree. The tree has not been created but is the result of a certain type of perception. It is only our perception that can vary and be subtler or grosser. Likewise, the universe was not created as we perceive it. We grasp reality according to what our senses reveal to us. The shape of the tree does not really exist as such; it is what our senses allow us to perceive. Therefore, the *Rig Veda* states:

एकं सद्विप्रा बहुधा वदन्ति ।

ekaṁ sad viprā bahudhā vadanti

Poets, sages, and masters call the one Being by different names.

(*Rig Veda,* 1.164.46)

And the *Śrīmad-bhāgavatam* says:

वदन्ति तत्तत्त्वविदस्तत्त्वं यज्ज्ञानमद्वयम् ।
ब्रह्मेति परमात्मेति भगवानिति शब्द्यते ॥

vadanti tat tattva-vidas
tattvaṁ yaj jñānam advayam
brahmeti paramātmeti
bhagavān iti śabdyate

The sages and seers who have realized the absolute Truth refer to the non-dual as Brahman, Paramātmā, or Bhagavān.

(*Śrīmad-bhāgavatam*, 1.2.11)

Undoubtedly, after eating or sleeping well, we experience a certain satisfaction or feeling of plenitude. However, it is not an absolute satisfaction; it is relative and temporary. The next day we will be hungry and sleepy again. Therefore, this is only a passing experience of happiness or satisfaction.

The realization of our original wholeness is only feasible after awakening to the awareness that subject and object, observer and observed, are one and the same. The difference we experience between subject and object is only apparent. Based on illusion, we isolate ourselves from life, identifying ourselves with an idea called "I." We observe the world from within a sack of flesh and bones with walls of skin, through the windows of the senses, and with the mind as the filter that evaluates what is perceived. We believe that what is perceived is completely different from the perceiver. We even believe that the mind–body complex is the perceiver. All that we consider perceivable through our senses is *idaṁ*, or what is generally called "manifested or material." The reality of the observer is no greater than that of the observed, for the reality of both is one and the same: Brahman. The very moment we succeed in perceiving the observer and the observed, the subject and the object, both are immediately transformed into the observed. The subject–object duality vanishes only when reality is simultaneously acknowledged. The scriptures, in their function as *pramāṇa*, show that such difference is only apparent and reveal the unity.

We can see the entire Vedantic perspective reflected in this mantra. Illusorily, we ascribe a greater reality to the subject than the perceived objects. However, the reality of the observing subject is not superior to the reality of the observed objects. As subjectivity that perceives the empirical reality, we are no more real than what is perceived. Our authentic nature is unbounded consciousness or *pūrṇam*. Both subject and objects share the same essential substance: consciousness. The apparent subject–object duality is only a projection upon *pūrṇam*, which does not affect it at all. Neither waves, humidity, nor tsunamis can affect the essential substance of water. The characteristic diversity of phenomenal reality lacks authentic substantiality, but it is only superimposed on reality. Our authentic nature is the immutable and formless reality where all difference dissolves. The apparent activity and multiplicity of the sea are only waves, bubbles, and currents that manifest temporarily in the infinite ocean of *pūrṇam*, incapable of disturbing or limiting it. The only permanent reality is the unlimited and infinite pure consciousness, Brahman, or *pūrṇam*.

Mantra 1

ॐ ईशा वास्यमिदꣳ सर्वं यत्किञ्च जगत्यां जगत् ।
तेन त्यक्तेन भुञ्जीथा मा गृधः कस्यस्विद्धनम् ॥

oṁ īśāvāsyam idaṁ sarvaṁ
yat kiñca jagatyāṁ jagat
tena tyaktena bhuñjīthā
mā gṛdhaḥ kasya svid dhanam

All this, be it living beings or inert matter, is wrapped up by the Lord. Therefore, enjoy renouncing worldly pleasures. Do not covet, since all wealth belongs to someone else.

Commentary:

Iśāvāsyam idam sarvaṁ

This Upanishad derives its name from the first word, *Īśa*. *Īśa* means "possessor" and is derived from the root *īś*, "to possess or control." Its theological meaning is "Supreme Being or Supreme Lord," or in Sanskrit: Īśvara. Īśvara is the supreme power that regulates everything. In the devotional terminology of *bhakti*, Īśvara would be the equivalent of the term "Lord." Although Brahman is the main subject of the Upanishads, it also mentions Īśvara, which is Brahman conceptualized through *māyā*. Just as time is eternity perceived by the mind, Īśvara is absolute consciousness conceived from an egoic perspective. Īśvara is the concept of a higher power, although its meaning varies in different schools of Hinduism. Īśvara is synonymous with absolute reality, but it can also refer to a personal god. According to the Vedanta, Truth can be conceived of in different ways:

1. The absolute aspect, or Brahman, as the ultimate reality or consciousness.
2. The cosmic aspect, or Īśvara, as the ruler of the various functions of creation, preservation, and destruction of the cosmos.
3. The aspect of the one sent into the world to fulfill different functions, or *avatāra*.

4. The aspect of the family deity, or *kula-devatā*.
5. The aspect of the deity favored by the devotee, or *iṣṭa-devatā*.

These different conceptions of divinity gradually become centered on the individual. They descend from the universal to the individual, leaving devotees to choose to adhere to a certain aspect of Truth according to their capabilities.

The term *Īśa* appears for the first time in the *Manu-smṛti*. In the *Śvetāśvatara Upanishad, Īśa* refers to Rudra. Shaivism uses this word as an integral part of the term Maheśvara, or "great Lord," to refer to Śiva. In Shaktism, on the other hand, the feminine term Īśvarī refers to the Divine Mother of the Universe. In fact, Īśvara is Brahman perceived from the dual and relative platform. The Lord envelops this universe in names and forms. Every living being is spirit or consciousness that appears to be wrapped in matter. God is the very essence of each one of us, as stated by the holy Bhagavad Gita:

सर्वस्य चाहं हृदि सन्निविष्टो मत्तः स्मृतिर्ज्ञानमपोहनञ्च ।
वेदैश्च सर्वैरहमेव वेद्यो वेदान्तकृद्वेदविदेव चाहम् ॥

sarvasya cāhaṁ hṛdi sanniviṣṭo
mattaḥ smṛtir jñānam apohanañ ca
vedaiś ca sarvair aham eva vedyo
vedānta-kṛd veda-vid eva cāham

> I am situated in everyone's heart, from me come remembrance, wisdom, and forgetfulness. I am the one to be known through all the Vedas. Truly, I am the compiler of Vedanta and the knower of the Vedas.
>
> (Bhagavad Gita, 15.15)

As explained in the commentary on the invocation, Brahman is the unlimited totality, which is revealed as the creator God (Īśvara) in the context of relative reality (*māyā*). Through the veil of ignorance (*avidyā*), Brahman itself is perceived in the form of innumerable souls (*jīvas*) who undergo the repeated cycle births and deaths because they do not know their divine nature. When perceiving Brahman through the veil of the *tamasic* aspect of *prakṛti*, *jīvas* see it as the manifested universe made up of the five subtle elements (*sūkṣma-bhūtas*). These elements form the mind, the intellect, the ego, the senses, life force, the organs of action, the body, and the gross elements (*sthūla-bhūtas*) that make up the diversity of the physical universe.

It is a grave mistake to think that *sanātana-dharma* is a polytheistic religion just because it believes in a plurality of gods. But neither can we categorize it as monotheistic, because its theology does not focus on a single God creator of the universe. According to the eternal dharma, only God is. The same truth is stated in the Hebrew Torah:

> אַתָּה הָרְאֵתָ לָדַעַת כִּי ה' הוּא הָאֱלֹהִים אֵין עוֹד מִלְבַדּוֹ.
> (דברים ד', ל"ה)

I have shown you and you have known that *Ha'shem* is God; there is nothing but Him.

(Deuteronomy, 4:35)

The Jewish Rabbi Ha Gaon Chayim of Volozhin (1749–1821) quotes the *Gemara* (*Chulin* page 7b), where it is taught:

אֵין עוֹד מִלְּבַדּוֹ. אָמַר רַבִּי חֲנִינָא: וַאֲפִילּוּ כְּשָׁפִים.
(תלמוד בבלי, חולין, דף ז', ע"ב)

"There is nothing but Him." Rabbi Hanina says: "And not even sorcery."

(*Talmud Bavli*, *Chulin*, 7b)

He then explains:

כְּשֶׁהָאָדָם קוֹבֵעַ בְּלִבּוֹ לֵאמֹר: הֲלֹא ה' הוּא הָאֱלֹקִים הָאֲמִתִּי וְאֵין עוֹד מִלְּבַדּוֹ יִתְבָּרֵךְ שׁוּם כֹּחַ בָּעוֹלָם וְכָל הָעוֹלָמוֹת כְּלָל וְהַכֹּל מָלֵא רַק אַחְדוּתוֹ הַפָּשׁוּט יִתְבָּרֵךְ שְׁמוֹ. וּמְבַטֵּל בְּלִבּוֹ בִּטּוּל גָּמוּר וְאֵינוֹ מַשְׁגִּיחַ כְּלָל עַל שׁוּם כֹּחַ וְרָצוֹן בָּעוֹלָם. וּמְשַׁעְבֵּד וּמְדַבֵּק טֹהַר מַחְשַׁבְתּוֹ רַק לָאָדוֹן יָחִיד בָּרוּךְ הוּא. כֵּן יַסְפִּיק הוּא יִתְבָּרֵךְ בְּיָדוֹ שֶׁמִּמֵּילָא יִתְבַּטְּלוּ מֵעָלָיו כָּל הַכֹּחוֹת וְהָרְצוֹנוֹת שֶׁבָּעוֹלָם שֶׁלֹּא יוּכְלוּ לִפְעֹל לוֹ שׁוּם דָּבָר כְּלָל.
(רבי חיים מוולוז'ין, נפש החיים, שער ג', פרק י"ב)

When a person fixes in one's heart that *Ha'shem* is the true God and there is no other power in the universe nor in any of all the worlds other than

> Him (Blessed be He), and everything is filled only with His (blessed be His name) absolute unity, and, in one's heart one completely nullifies and does not regard any power or will in the universe, and one harnesses and adheres one's pure thoughts only to the one Lord (blessed is He), then divine He, blessed be him, will grant that person, as a natural consequence, that all the powers and desires that are in the universe will be nullified before that person, so that they will not be able to affect him or her in any way at all. (Rabbi Chaim of Volozhin, *Nefesh Ha'chayim*, 3.12)

"Therefore, enjoy renouncing worldly pleasures."

Many people might mistakenly think that renouncing means decreasing our capacity for happiness or enjoyment. Quite the contrary, attachments impede bliss. All addictions hinder access to true happiness. *Tena tyaktena bhuñjīthā* means "enjoy renouncing," because every attachment brings an impurity that restricts our freedom. Only those who love shall discover the pleasure of renouncing. Only those who love animals will enjoy renouncing eating meat. Only those who love life will enjoy renouncing drugs. Only those who love other human beings will enjoy renouncing part of their bread to share it with the hungry. Only those who love us will be happy to sacrifice for our well-being. Without love, we only recognize pleasure when we receive or consume something. Only those who walk in love live in this world as contributors. Only love allows us to willingly renounce our personal enjoyment for the benefit of others. Only those who love enjoy effort, sacrifice, and renouncing. Only those who love God know the enjoyment of renouncing themselves and their selfishness.

If we observe ourselves through a limited mind and imperfect senses, we feel confined by the limits of time and space. Believing ourselves to be a separate subject, disconnected from the objective world, we feel something is missing. When we perceive our own limitations, the feelings of scarcity, restriction, discomfort, disconnection, and insufficiency emerge. Our ability for self-observation induces a deep dissatisfaction and uneasiness because we feel confined in physical bodies and endowed with limited knowledge. We try to complete ourselves with the objective world, finding only frustration in the end. This disappointment is due to the fact that nothing and no one can complete us, because we are already complete. By renouncing our efforts to achieve happiness and security through the objective world, we shall enjoy without disappointment. Renouncing the inclination to try to complete ourselves is a sign of spiritual maturity.

The mantra calls for renouncing our efforts to complete ourselves through empirical reality. Along with maturity comes the realization that the satisfaction of our desires lacks permanence. At different stages of life, our objects of pleasure vary. Children delight in objects that are very different from those of teens or adults. During childhood, we enjoy toys; during youth, music; in our adulthood, family. However, our sense that something is missing remains throughout life. Pleasures may change, but our deep sense of absence does not. Worldly enjoyments are limited by time and space, while our true longing is for eternal and absolute bliss. Thus, the egoic phenomenon is the experience of lack or scarcity. The idea of "I" resembles a very deep hole that each one carries within oneself and that is impossible to fill. Throughout our lives, we strive to throw heavy stones into the hole in the form of money, jewelry, objects, people, fame, honor, and so on, but yet it remains empty. On the contrary, the more we try to plug the egoic hole, the wider it gets.

Unhappiness, sadness, and pain revolve around the idea of "I." The egoic phenomenon is the source and foundation for all dissatisfaction. Therefore, we can affirm that the original unqualified desire is the desire to complete oneself and to remove the sense of limitation. This is the original desire from which all desires are born and originate. Trying to free ourselves from the deep feeling of limitation, we focus our efforts on searching for objects, in the hope of experiencing fullness and totality. We experience a wide variety of desires and unfailingly all of them originate in our sense of absence. A feeling of vulnerability motivates our search for security. Suffering prompts us to seek happiness. Our need for love is born out of loneliness. This experience of deficiency is the origin of our desires. Motivated by it, we strive to complete ourselves by satisfying our mental demands on the objective plane.

Our original nature of unlimited bliss prompts us to seek happiness and avoid suffering. We are constantly trying to escape the uncomfortable situation of feeling constrained by a form. Nothing and no one in the objective world can free us from the pursuit of pleasure and enjoyment. This destitution is inherent in our slavery. Instead of condemning efforts to satisfy the senses, Vedanta focuses on a deep understanding of the nature of desire. It does not suggest a blind and ignorant repression of desires, but a liberation from constantly pursuing them.

आपूर्यमाणमचलप्रतिष्ठं समुद्रमापः प्रविशन्ति यद्वत् ।
तद्वत्कामा यं प्रविशन्ति सर्वे स शान्तिमाप्नोति न कामकामी ॥

āpūryamāṇam acala-pratiṣṭhaṁ
samudram āpaḥ praviśanti yadvat
tadvat kāmā yaṁ praviśanti sarve
sa śāntim āpnoti na kāma-kāmī

Just as innumerable rivers flow in the ocean, which is full and remains calm, peace can be attained only by those who remains undisturbed despite the various desires flowing into their mind; but not by those who always strive to satisfy their desires.

(Bhagavad Gita, 2.70)

विहाय कामान्यः सर्वान्पुमांश्चरति निःस्पृहः ।
निर्ममो निरहङ्कारः स शान्तिमधिगच्छति ॥

vihāya kāmān yaḥ sarvān
pumāṁś carati niḥspṛhaḥ
nirmamo nirahaṅkāraḥ
sa śāntim adhigacchati

Peace is achieved by the person who, abandoning all desires, moves without anxiety, without sense of self, and without selfishness.

(Bhagavad Gita, 2.71)

एषा ब्राह्मी स्थितिः पार्थ नैनां प्राप्य विमुह्यति ।
स्थित्वास्यामन्तकालेऽपि ब्रह्मनिर्वाणमृच्छति ॥

eṣā brāhmī sthitiḥ pārtha
naināṁ prāpya vimuhyati
sthitvāsyām anta-kāle 'pi
brahma-nirvāṇam ṛcchati

This is the Brahminic state (eternal state), O son of Pṛthā! After attaining this state, one is no longer deluded. Being established in that state, even at the end of life, one reaches oneness with Brahman.

(Bhagavad Gita, 2.72)

The bliss of the enlightened sages does not depend on the pleasure that the phenomenal world bestows on them. While the desire of the ordinary person is born from a feeling of lack, the desire of the wise ones emerges from plenitude. As a result, although they have desires, they are not bound by them, and thus, they do not enslave, chain, or tie them down.

When a binding desire is not satisfied, it causes discomfort. Ordinary human beings enjoy satisfying their desires and are frustrated when they cannot. For someone who is enlightened, everything is perception or consciousness; therefore, desires do not originate from absence or scarcity. There are many who ignorantly condemn desires and strive to repress them. But enlightened sages understand that the problem is not desire itself, but its relation with objects. Their desires lack goals since they are not related to objects; thus, they experience pure desire, free of all motivation.

Nothing and no one can satisfy our desires. With such clear understanding, sages stop desiring objects or people and live flowing in desire at all times. Living in desire, life fills with passion. Enlightened beings constantly rest in their true blissful nature, regardless of whether or not they obtain sensory enjoyment. If pleasure manifests itself, they will enjoy it, but if not, the absence of pleasure will not cloud their transcendental bliss. Recognizing themselves as consciousness itself, they do not seek to be completed by anything or anyone.

Intensely enjoy the pleasure you may find on your

path, but do not try to repeat it. Enjoy the present without trying to clone yesterday. The pleasure you find on your path today is a gift of existence, so enjoy it! When your mind interferes and you think of that pleasure, the desire and the attempt to repeat it awaken. The memory of that pleasure becomes a force in your life. Without realizing it, you seek to duplicate the same situation and the same tastes. The memory of past pleasures induces you to reproduce them, creating chains that enslave you. This is where attachments and addictions are born. Live in the present and enjoy the now.

"Do not covet, since all wealth belongs to someone else."

The sage advises us to not covet. Greed is born in hearts motivated by possessiveness. We mistakenly believe that our situation will improve if we only had more. However, we do not understand that our misery, loneliness, and conditioning will not change with having more of what we already have. Our misery will not cease by gathering more money, alcohol, fame, honor, or possessions. If I am unhappy with my belongings, it is not very smart to covet more of the same. The required change is not quantitative but qualitative. What is required is to turn on our inner light. What we need is a qualitative transformation at the level of consciousness.

Greed is another way of deferring the present: postponing life in order to live in a hypothetical future.

Only those who are free of greed can place themselves in the present and experience life in all its intensity.

It is inappropriate to call something a *possession* if it must be returned later. What must be repaid should be called a *loan*, not a possession. We can use the term *possession* for what is ours that we will never have to give back to anyone. If we think about what we consider to be "our possessions," we will see that sooner or later we will have to return them all. Human beings claim to own their bodies, the sea, the sky and the earth, which is obviously ridiculous. Humans, who hardly live 80 or 90 years, cannot own a piece of land that was there long before they were born and will continue there long after they return their bodies to the Lord. If we lived according to this truth, we would begin to love others for who they are and not for what they have. Sooner or later, we will all have to separate from what we consider our possessions. Thus, "all wealth that belongs to someone else" only belongs to the Lord. If we reason about the temporality of the body and our so-called possessions, we will be able to observe life with greater maturity. Such a perspective will help us live a more authentic life.

Mantra 2

कुर्वन्नेवेह कर्माणि जिजीविषेच्छतं समाः ।
एवं त्वयि नान्यथेतोऽस्ति न कर्म लिप्यते नरे ॥

kurvann eveha karmāṇi
jijīviṣec chataṁ samāḥ
evaṁ tvayi nānyatheto 'sti
na karma lipyate nare

Acting in the world in accordance with this wisdom, one can aspire to live a hundred years, without action restricting one's freedom.

Commentary:

In order to understand this verse, we first need to explore the basics of the yoga of action, or karma yoga, and understand what action is and how it restricts our freedom.

The Sanskrit word *karma* means "action." It is derived from the Sanskrit root *kri*, which means "to do or to act." The term is also used in Buddhism, Jainism, and later in spiritism. Karma refers to both "action or activity" and its "result or effect." Virtually everyone has heard of the law of karma or the law of cause and effect. In physics, the term is equivalent to Newton's third law of motion: "For every action there is an equal and opposite reaction." The principle of the law of karma states that the intentions and actions of each individual will influence their future.

Every action brings about a reaction, originating in a merit or demerit with its corresponding fruits in the present or next life. As the *Devī-bhāgavatam* states:

याद‍ृशं कुरुते कर्म ताद‍ृशं फलमाप्नुयात् ।
अवश्यमेव भोक्तव्यं कृतं कर्म शुभाशुभम् ॥

yādṛśaṁ kurute karma
tādṛśaṁ phalam āpnuyāt
avaśyam eva bhoktavyaṁ
kṛtaṁ karma śubhāśubham

> In accordance with the work (karma) being done, so will be the fruits that are obtained. The effects of karma must be harvested whether they are auspicious or inauspicious.
>
> (*Devī-bhāgavatam*, 6.9.67)

Cause and effect are inseparable. The effect lies in potential form within the cause, which, in turn, manifests as the effect. Within the seed lies the potential tree; the tree is the manifestation of the seed.

Vedantic wisdom affirms that the entire universe is under the control of this infallible and absolute law from which it is impossible to escape. The law of karma governs all movement, from atoms and cells to galaxies and universes, and it encompasses all they contain, visible and invisible.

In the *Śrīmad-devī-bhāgavatam*, Vyāsadeva tells King Janamejaya:

उत्पत्तिः सर्वजन्तूनां विना कर्म न विद्यते ।
कर्मणा भ्रमते सूर्यः शशाङ्कः क्षयरोगवान् ॥
कपाली च तथा रुद्रः कर्मणैव न संशयः ।
अनादिनिधनं चैतत्कारणं कर्म विद्यते ॥

utpattiḥ sarva-jantūnāṁ
vinā karma na vidyate
karmaṇā bhramate sūryaḥ
śaśāṅkaḥ kṣaya-rogavān

kapālī ca tathā rudraḥ
karmaṇaiva na saṁśayaḥ
anādi-nidhanaṁ caitat
kāraṇaṁ karma vidyate

O king, no creature can arise without karma. It is through karma that the sun traverses the sky; it is through karma that the moon was attacked with tuberculosis; and there is no doubt that through karma, Rudra holds the skull disc. This karma, therefore, has neither beginning nor end [until liberation], for this karma is the sole cause in the production of this universe.

(*Śrīmad-devī-bhāgavatam*, 4.2.12–13)

Any activity, be it physical, verbal, emotional, or mental, will produce a result, which can be positive or negative. Wherever there is action, a reaction is inevitable. Our present life is conditioned by activities carried out in past lives, and our current activities will influence future lives.

Studying the law of karma, we understand the great responsibility that we have to our own destiny. We have complete freedom to choose how we act and later, we will suffer or enjoy the consequences of our choices. These reactions keep us enslaved to this relative world and are the cause of our reincarnation, life after life.

Generally, we strive to obtain specific results in life. If the results of our work are pleasing, we accept them and take the corresponding credit. On the other hand, when the natural consequences of our actions are painful, we deny our participation in the causes. Then we simply attribute responsibility to external factors and circumstances. Through the law of karma, we understand that we are the architects of our own destiny. Karma yoga is the path that leads us to transcend the consequences, both pleasing and painful, of our actions.

This concept leads us to take responsibility for the consequences of our actions. It demands we are more aware of what we do and the motivations for our behavior. For example, the following Baha'í teachings refer to the consequences of negative actions, as well as the importance of being aware of them:

> O companion of my throne! Hear no evil, and see no evil, abase not thyself, neither sigh and weep. Speak no evil, that thou mayest not hear it spoken unto thee, and magnify not the faults of others that thine own faults may not appear great; and wish not the abasement of anyone, that thine own abasement be not exposed. Live then the days of thy life, that are less than a fleeting moment, with thy mind stainless, thy heart unsullied, thy thoughts pure, and thy nature sanctified, so that, free and content, thou mayest put away this mortal frame, and repair unto the mystic paradise and abide in the eternal kingdom for evermore.
>
> (*Bahá'u'lláh*, *The Hidden Words*, 44)

The Jewish *Mishnah* narrates a story about Hillel the elder, which presents a similar concept:

> אַף הוּא רָאָה גֻּלְגֹּלֶת אַחַת שֶׁצָּפָה עַל פְּנֵי הַמָּיִם. אָמַר לָהּ: עַל דַּאֲטֵפְתְּ, אַטְפוּךְ; וְסוֹף מְטַיְּפַיִךְ יְטוּפוּן.
> (פרקי אבות ב', ו')
>
> Moreover, he saw a skull floating on the surface of the water. He said to it: "because you drowned others, others will drown you. And in the end, those who drowned you will be drowned."
>
> (*Pirkei Avot*, 2.6)

Throughout life, we face various tests that evaluate us. Problematic results are created by our weaknesses and it is our successes that give us a certain well-being. Our activities influence us as much or even more than we influence them. Both by harming and benefiting other beings, we harm and benefit ourselves. As the *Bṛhad-āraṇyaka Upanishad* points out:

> **तद्यदेतदिदंमयोऽदोमय इति; यथाकारी यथाचारी तथा भवति— साधुकारी साधुर्भवति, पापकारी पापो भवति; पुण्यः पुण्येन कर्मणा भवति, पापः पापेन ।**
>
> *tad yad etad idaṁ mayo 'do maya iti; yathā kārī yathā cārī tathā bhavati— sādhu-kārī sādhur bhavati, pāpa-kārī pāpo bhavati; puṇyaḥ puṇyena karmaṇā bhavati, pāpaḥ pāpena.*

> The embodied soul becomes what it does and how it acts; by doing good it becomes good, and by doing evil it becomes evil—it becomes virtuous through good acts and vicious through evil acts.
>
> (*Bṛhad-āraṇya Upanishad*, 4.4.5)

Vedanta considers life to be a great school for the soul, in which we develop and evolve through different situations. In this context, the law of karma, applied consciously, fulfills a very important function whose purpose is not to punish but to educate.

The path of karma yoga leads us to liberation from karma and the wheel of *saṁsāra.* At its highest stage, it guides us to the direct realization that there is not—and never was—a cause producing an effect. The apparent separation between cause and effect is only a mental creation. The mind perceives fruits as the fulfilment of work. Thc cgoic phcnomcnon trics to scc thc culmination of action in the results. It strives in the present with the aim of perpetuating itself through effect in the future. In reality, cause and effect are one. The division between acts and results is nothing more than the product of the mind.

The *guṇas*

During their lives, human beings inevitably experience dark periods of turmoil in which they feel lost. They have times of laziness, weaknesses, and addiction when they lack the energy to resist fears and do not know what to do or which direction to take. Likewise, almost no one is exempt from moments of rage, anger, aggression, and violence. There are also days filled with the desire to sacrifice for something worthy of our effort. People also enjoy blissful moments of introspection, in which they experience clarity, inexplicable calm, and peace. *Sāṅkhya* philosophy teaches us that the reason for these different states is found in the *tri-guṇa,* or "the three modes of nature."

Knowledge about the *guṇas* is essential for anyone who wants to understand the path of karma yoga. In the Bhagavad Gita, Lord Kṛṣṇa refers to this as follows:

सत्त्वं रजस्तम इति गुणाः प्रकृतिसम्भवाः ।
निबध्नन्ति महाबाहो देहे देहिनमव्ययम् ॥

sattvaṁ rajas tama iti
guṇāḥ prakṛti-sambhavāḥ
nibadhnanti mahā-bāho
dehe dehinam avyayam

O Arjuna, the one with powerful arms, the primordial nature consists of three *guṇas*: harmony (*sattva*), passion (*rajas*), and inertia (*tamas*), which enslave the immutable embodied being.

(Bhagavad Gita, 14.5)

The *prakṛti-śakti,* or "creative power," of Brahman

comprises three qualities (*guṇas*) that act interdependently: *tamas* (laziness or inertia), *rajas* (passion), and *sattva* (goodness or harmony). These modes constitute the substance from which the universe emanates. All that exists, both mental and physical, is nothing but the result of different combinations of the three *guṇas*. Any distinction that we perceive between objects, places or human beings is due to these modalities, which combine and interact as part of the evolution of *prakṛti*.

Tamas is the mode of ignorance, laziness, and drowsiness. *Tamas* delays and obstructs action, induces negligence, and keeps consciousness obscured. Usually, the motivations for tamasic activities are gross sensory enjoyment and escape from immediate discomfort. The Bhagavad Gita refers to the mode of ignorance as follows:

तमस्त्वज्ञानजं विद्धि मोहनं सर्वदेहिनाम् ।
प्रमादालस्यनिद्राभिस्तन्निबध्नाति भारत ॥

tamas tvajñāna-jaṁ viddhi
mohanaṁ sarva-dehinām
pramādālasya-nidrābhis
tan nibadhnāti bhārata

O son of Bharata! Know that the inertia of *tamas*, born of ignorance, leads to confusion and binds embodied beings through negligence, laziness, and sleep.

(Bhagavad Gita, 14.8)

Rajas is the mode of passion that creates conflict and turbulence. Rajasic actions tend to disrupt balance and harmony, ultimately leading to disintegration. Rajasic actions are externalized, always pursue a result, and try to demonstrate, promote, or feign something. *Rajas* induces us to be attached to the result of our actions. Typically, the motivations of rajasic activities are attachment, power, fame, and wealth. The Bhagavad Gita refers to the mode of passion as follows:

रजो रागात्मकं विद्धि तृष्णासङ्गसमुद्भवम् ।
तन्निबध्नाति कौन्तेय कर्मसङ्गेन देहिनम् ॥

rajo rāgātmakaṁ viddhi
tṛṣṇā-saṅga-samudbhavam
tan nibadhnāti kaunteya
karma-saṅgena dehinam

Know, O son of Kuntī, that *rajas*, the mode of passion, is born of desire and attachment. This binds the embodied being through attachment to action.

(Bhagavad Gita, 14.7)

Finally, *sattva* is the mode of goodness, virtue, clarity, and intelligence. Sattvic actions tend to harmonize, balance, and internalize us. Although all the modes of nature keep the soul enslaved, *sattva* is the one that provides the best opportunity to transcend. When this modality is prevalent in our lives, we have a greater chance of realizing transcendental consciousness. The Bhagavad Gita refers to the mode of goodness as follows:

तत्र सत्त्वं निर्मलत्वात्प्रकाशकमनामयम् ।
सुखसङ्गेन बध्नाति ज्ञानसङ्गेन चानघ ॥

tatra sattvaṁ nirmalatvāt
prakāśakam anāmayam
sukha-saṅgena badhnāti
jñāna-saṅgena cānagha

> O, you, the immaculate one!, the mode of goodness, being of higher purity than the rest, illuminates and heals. It binds through attachment to happiness and knowledge.
> (Bhagavad Gita, 14.6)

The *guṇas* are experienced through our emotional and sentimental movement, that is to say, through psychological activity. We tend to believe that we are the doers who freely decide what to do or what not to do in our lives. However, in reality, we do not act with free will, but according to the modality of nature that is imposed at a given moment or situation. These three modalities are always present in every human being: always one predominates over the others. As the Bhagavad Gita goes on to point out:

रजस्तमश्चाभिभूय सत्त्वं भवति भारत ।
रजः सत्त्वं तमश्चैव तमः सत्त्वं रजस्तथा ॥

rajas tamaś cābhibhūya
sattvaṁ bhavati bhārata
rajaḥ sattvaṁ tamaś caiva
tamaḥ sattvam rajas tathā

At certain times, harmony (*sattva*) predominates over passion (*rajas*). At other times, it is passion (*rajas*) that predominates over inertia (*tamas*) and harmony, and sometimes it is inertia that predominates over harmony and passion.

(Bhagavad Gita, 14.10)

When *tamas* is the predominant *guṇa*, people are characterized by lethargy and indolence. They do not act logically and are not guided by reason. Their actions are instinctive; they do what they like to do and postpone what they do not.

When *rajas* is the predominant *guṇa*, people plan, program, and assess. They feel compelled to act. On the other hand, when *sattva* is prevalent, they are calm and serene. It is not possible for a tamasic person to suddenly reach the sattvic level. The changes are gradual and organic. *Tamas* can turn into *rajas* and *rajas* into *sattva*. This is described in the Bhagavad Gita:

सर्वद्वारेषु देहेऽस्मिन्प्रकाश उपजायते ।
ज्ञानं यदा तदा विद्याद्विवृद्धं सत्त्वमित्युत ॥
लोभः प्रवृत्तिरारम्भः कर्मणामशमः स्पृहा ।
रजस्येतानि जायन्ते विवृद्धे भरतर्षभ ॥
अप्रकाशोऽप्रवृत्तिश्च प्रमादो मोह एव च ।
तमस्येतानि जायन्ते विवृद्धे कुरुनन्दन ॥

sarva-dvāreṣu dehe 'smin
prakāśa upajāyate
jñānaṁ yadā tadā vidyād
vivṛddhaṁ sattvam ity uta

lobhaḥ pravṛttir ārambhaḥ
karmaṇām aśamaḥ spṛhā
rajasy etāni jāyante
vivṛddhe bharata-ṛṣabha

aprakāśo 'pravṛttiś ca
pramādo moha eva ca
tamasy etāni jāyante
vivṛddhe kuru-nandana

O Arjuna, when, through every portal (every sense) in this body, the light of wisdom shines, then it may be known that *sattva* is predominant. When *rajas* is predominant, greed, activity, undertaking actions, restlessness, and longing arise. When *tamas* is predominant, darkness, inertia, negligence, and delusion arise.

(Bhagavad Gita, 14.11–13)

The action's process

Whenever we try to achieve a purpose, there is a process of knowledge (*jñāna*). This leads to a desire or feeling (*cikīrṣā* or *icchā*) and then to a will to act (*pravṛtti*), which causes a motor effect (*ceṣṭā*), and finally action (*kārya*) occurs.

Udayanācārya describes this in the *Nyāya-kusumāñjalī*:

प्रवृत्तिः कृतिरेवात्र सा चेच्छातो यतश्च स ।
तज्ज्ञानं विषयस्तस्य विधिस्तज्ज्ञापकोऽथ वा ॥

pravṛttiḥ kṛtir evātra
sā cecchāto yataś ca sā
taj jñānaṁ viṣayas tasya
vidhis taj jñāpako 'thavā

The action (*pravṛtti*) here is the effort (*kṛti* or *kriyā*) itself and it arises due to a feeling or desire (*icchā*). The feeling arises from knowledge (*jñāna*) and the object of this knowledge is said to be the command (*vidhi*), or it is rather that which causes the command to be inferred.

(*Nyāya-kusumāñjalī*, 5.7)

This process is also mentioned in the *Śrī-caitanya-caritāmṛta*, regarding the cosmic creation:

ইচ্ছাজ্ঞানক্রিয়া ৱিনা না হয সৃজন ।
তিনের তিনশক্তি মেলি' প্রপঞ্চরচন ॥

icchā-jñāna-kriyā vinā nā haya sṛjana
tinera tina-śakti meli' prapañca-racana

There is no possibility of creation without feeling, knowledge, and activity. The combination of these three powers brings about the cosmic manifestation.

(*Śrī-caitanya-caritāmṛta*, "*Mādhya-līlā*," 20.254)

- *Jnāna* or "knowledge": All activities are expressions of thought and come from ideas. Knowledge is thought, memory, and the past.
- *Cikīrṣā* or "desire": Knowledge (*jñāna*) of an object leads to a feeling of attraction or rejection toward it. If it has caused us pleasant experiences, we will want to repeat them and desire (*icchā*) will be born. If it causes us painful experiences, fear will arise.
- *Pravṛtti* or "will to act": Out of attraction or rejection, there emerges a will to perform certain actions. *Pravṛtti* is a Sanskrit term that means "go toward" or "revolve around external elements."
- *Ceṣṭā* or "motor effect": The will to act gives rise to the effort to obtain or remove an object.
- *Kārya* or "action": Finally, action follows. Immersed in this process, our actions are not free;

> they are conditioned by desire and fear. Karma is the result of the process that comprises all of the factors mentioned above. A life chained to action will always be linear because we are drawn in a single direction. We believe we are free and we pursue happiness or escape from suffering. The only possible choice is to do it on foot, by bicycle, or in a car. Furthermore, someone considered successful in our society is not freer but only has the economic means to afford a private jet. Therefore, our actions may become more sophisticated, but our slavery keeps us internally stagnant.

Knowledge is like the seed, desire the tree, and action the fruit. Therefore, every action is a projection of the desire that originated it and the manifestation on the gross level of movements on much subtler levels. Even the legal system judges not only actions, but also the intention and attitude of the accused, that is, the thoughts that preceded the action. For example, the punishment for premeditated murder is much more severe than involuntary manslaughter.

Positive and inspiring actions arise from benevolent and elevated desires, while negative actions stem from perverse ambitions and destructive intentions.

We find expression for these ideas in the four castes of Vedic society, which are distinguished according to their motivation. The motivation of the *śūdra* is sensual pleasure; *vaiśya*, riches; *kṣatriya*, power; and *brāhmaṇa*,

God. *Śūdras* act out of fear, *vaiśyas* and *kṣatriyas* out of a desire for gain, and *brāhmaṇas* out of inspiration.

Just as attitude influences activity, our motivations influence us. It is thus essential to feed our mind with elevated thoughts to purify the desires that enslave us and convert those desires into liberating aspirations.

Types of karma

1. Negative, positive, and combined karma

The sage Patañjali Maharṣi writes in *Yoga Sūtra* that karma can be negative, positive, or combined.

> कर्माशुक्लाकृष्णं योगिनस्त्रिविधमितरेषाम् ॥
>
> *karmāśuklākṛṣṇaṁ yoginas tri-vidham itareṣām*
>
> For the yogi, karma is neither black nor white; for others it can be one of three types: white, black, or combined.
>
> (*Yoga Sūtra*, 4.7)

1.1 Negative karma

> तत्र कृष्णा दुरात्मनाम् ।
>
> *tatra kṛṣṇā durātmanām.*

> There, black (karma) is the sinful one.
>
> (*Yoga-sūtra-bhāṣya of Vyāsa* on *Yoga Sūtra* 4.7)

Negative reactions are generated by activities that damage, injure, and create separation. One who acts violently and aggressively, humiliates and offends others, and causes pain should not be surprised if the response is equally hostile. Lord Ṛṣabha explains to his sons:

नूनं प्रमत्तः कुरुते विकर्म यदिन्द्रियप्रीतय आपृणोति ।
न साधु मन्ये यत आत्मनोऽयमसन्नपि क्लेशद आस देहः ॥

nūnaṁ pramattaḥ kurute vikarma
yad indriya-prītaya āpṛṇoti
na sādhu manye yata ātmano 'yam
asann api kleśa-da āsa dehaḥ

> Indeed, I believe that it is not proper of the soul the mad person who performs undesirable acts for the satisfaction of the senses. These acts caused the temporary existence of the body, which is the source of suffering.
>
> (*Śrīmad-bhāgavatam*, 5.5.4)

On more subtle levels of thought and feeling, a depressive attitude toward life produces negative karma. Searching for the weaknesses and faults of others, judging and condemning them can lead to depression, psychological disorders and mental illness. The result of negative karma will be a birth into a lower form of life. Evil actions lead to degradation in spiritual evolution.

1.2. Positive karma

वेदप्रणिहितो धर्मः कर्म यन्मङ्गलं परम् ।
अवैदिकं तु यत्कर्म तदेवाशुभमेव च ॥

veda-praṇihito dharmaḥ
karma yan maṅgalaṁ param
avaidikaṁ tu yat karma
tad evāśubham eva ca

The karma that the Vedas say leads to dharma is good; all other actions are bad.

(*Devī-bhāgavatam*, 9.28.5)

Positive karma consists of good actions. However, one should not confuse good or charitable actions with karma yoga. Although goodness elevates us and transforms us into celestial beings, it can only lead to happiness, not transcendental bliss. Good actions can bring us positive karma, but in karma yoga, we transcend all results. *Karma-yogīs* are not "good" but transcendental, because they do not create good karma; they renounce it completely.

Philanthropy and volunteer work for charitable organizations is not necessarily karma yoga. Not every action that seems beneficial can be called karma yoga.

Throughout history, tyrants and dictators have considered the murder of millions of people to be a service to humanity. Nuclear weapons are developed by world powers in the belief that it serves their national interest. Out of ignorance, what seems beneficial may be nothing more than a misguided whim that only causes damage and harm.

This is so true that the sage Vyāsa, in his commentary to the *Yoga Sūtra*, says that all external actions produce combined karma; only inner activities are purely positive.

> शुक्ला तपःस्वाध्यायध्यानवताम् । सा हि केवले मनस्यायत्तत्वाद बहिःसाधनाधिना न परांपीडयित्वा भवति ।
>
> *śuklā tapaḥ-svādhyāya-dhyānavatām. sā hi kevale manasyāyat tatvāda-bahiḥ sādhanādhinā na parān pīḍayitvā bhavati.*
>
> White karma belongs to those who surrender themselves to penance, study, and contemplation; these activities, being confined solely to the mind, cannot be performed externally, and as such, cannot inflict pain on others.
>
> (*Yoga-sūtra-bhāṣya of Vyāsa* on *Yoga Sūtra* 4.7)

Moreover, any activity or effort projected by a mental idea cannot be karma yoga. Only service approved by the Vedic scriptures and in compliance with the specific order of our spiritual master is truly karma yoga.

1.3. Combined karma

शुक्लकृष्णा बहिः साधनसाध्या । तत्र परपीडानुग्रहद्वारेणैव कर्माशयप्रचयः ॥

śukla-kṛṣṇā bahiḥ sādhana-sādhyā. tatra parapīḍānugraha-dvāreṇaiva karmāśaya-pracayaḥ.

White–black is accomplished by external means. Hence the accumulation of a latent store of karma is caused by injury and kindness to others.
(*Yoga-sūtra-bhāṣya of Vyāsa* on *Yoga Sūtra* 4.7)

Combined or mixed karma is actions that have a mixture of positive and negative karma. Mixed karma can be both beneficial and harmful, such as for example, stealing to buy medicine or food for the poor, or building a hospital with illegally-obtained funds.

We tend to encounter mixed karma in daily life, because in reality, actions are never completely good or completely bad. In every negative action, goodness is concealed, just as in any positive action, there is something negative. When we talk about action we are speaking of the relative world and setting foot on the dual terrain of the mind.

Positive karma is like a precious metal such as gold or platinum; mixed karma, a less expensive metal, such as silver; and negative karma, a cheap metal. However, it matters little what metal was used to make the bars of the cell that restricts our freedom. It is not the quality of the chains that is responsible for our suffering, but the chains themselves. If we continue to create karma—whether positive, negative, or mixed—we will continue to be chained to this world of birth, sickness, old age, and death. As long as our actions are only an escape from the disagreeable and a pursuit of the agreeable, our enslavement to karma will continue.

2. Past, present, and future karma

According to the sacred scriptures, there are three classes of karma:

कर्मणस्तु त्रिधा प्रोक्ता गतिस्तत्त्वविदां वरैः ।
सञ्चितं वर्तमानं च प्रारब्धमिति भेदतः ॥

karmaṇas tu tridhā proktā
gatis tattva-vidāṁ varaiḥ
sañcitaṁ vartamānaṁ ca
prārabdham iti bhedataḥ

It is said by the best knowers of the Truth that karma is divided into three kinds, accumulated (*sañcita*), present (*vartamāna*), and commenced (*prārabdha*).

(*Devī-bhāgavatam*, 6.10.8)

The sage Sūta explains to Śaunaka in the *Garuḍa Purāṇa*:

आचोद्यमानानि यथा पुष्पाणि च फलानि च ।
स्वकालं नातिवर्तन्ते तथा कर्म पुराकृतम् ॥

ācodyamānāni yathā
puṣpāṇi ca phalāni ca
svakālaṁ nātivartante
tathā karma purā-kṛtam

Flowers bloom and fruits ripen in their due time and of their own accord without waiting for anyone's bidding; the effects of one's karma also bide their time and only become manifest at the right time.

(*Garuḍa Purāṇa*, 1.113.51)

शीलं कुलं नैव न चैव विद्या ज्ञानं गुणा नैव न बीजशुद्धिः ।
भाग्यानि पूर्वं तपसार्जितानि काले फलन्त्यस्य यथैव वृक्षाः ॥

śīlaṁ kulaṁ naiva na caiva vidyā
jñānaṁ guṇā naiva na bīja-śuddhiḥ
bhāgyāni pūrvaṁ tapasārjitāni
kāle phalanty asya yathaiva vṛkṣāḥ

Character, birth, education, knowledge, conduct, virtue, and connection do not avail a person in this life. The effects of one's karma and penance, done in a previous existence, come to fruition like a tree at the appointed time, in the next existence.

(*Garuḍa Purāṇa*, 1.113.52)

तत्र मृत्युर्यत्र हन्ता तत्र श्रीर्यत्र सम्पदः ।
तत्र तत्र स्वयं याति प्रेर्यमाणः स्वकर्मभिः ॥

tatra mṛtyur yatra hantā
tatra śrīr yatra sampadaḥ
tatra tatra svayaṁ yāti
preryamāṇaḥ sva-karmabhiḥ

Wherever there is death, there is killing, wherever there is a good fortune, there is prosperity. Peoples' karma forcibly pulls them to the place where death or fortune awaits.

(*Garuḍa Purāṇa*, 1.113.53)

भूतपूर्वं कृतं कर्म कर्तारमनुतिष्ठति ।
यथा धेनुसहस्रेषु वत्सो विन्दन्ति मातरम् ॥

bhūta-pūrvaṁ kṛtaṁ karma
kartāram anutiṣṭhati
yathā dhenu-sahasreṣu
vatso vindanti mātaram

The effects of deeds (karma) done by people in a prior existence overtake and choose them in the next, as a calf finds its mother among a thousand cows.

(*Garuḍa Purāṇa*, 1.113.54)

एवं पूर्वकृतं कर्म कर्तारमनुतिष्ठाति ।
सुकृतं भुङ्क्ष्व चात्मीयं मूढ किं परितप्यसे ॥
यथा पूर्वकृतं कर्म शुभं वा यदि वाशुभम् ।
तथा जन्मान्तरे तद्वै कर्ता रमनुगच्छति ॥

evaṁ pūrva-kṛtaṁ karma
kartāram anutiṣṭhāti
sukṛtaṁ bhuṅkṣva cātmīyaṁ
mūḍha kiṁ paritapyase

yathā pūrva-kṛtaṁ karma
śubhaṁ vā yadi vāśubham
tathā janmāntare tad vai
kartāram anugacchati

Thus, people's karma binds them for good or for evil. Pleasure or pain and happiness or misery are the direct result of one's good or bad deeds in a prior life. Why do you make such a heavy stock of misery out of it, O foolish one?

(*Garuḍa Purāṇa*, 1,113.55–56)

2.1. *Sañcita-karma* or "karma accumulated in the past"

This is the sum total of all our past karma, the activities and results of all our past lives: what has been and what remains unmanifested. It is our total accumulated debt in the cosmic bank. Most of us continuously increase our *sañcita-karma* through current activities. Our personality, tendencies, inclinations, and talents are determined by part of our *sañcita-karma*.

For most of us, this is probably not the first time that we have occupied a human body. Perhaps many of us have had hundreds, thousands, or millions of human births on this planet. *Sañcita-karma* is the accumulation of all that we have thought, felt, said, or done, throughout all these lives.

The sixth book of the *Devī-bhāgavatam* (10.9–11) describes this type of karma.

अनेक-जन्म-सञ्जातं प्राक्तनं सञ्चितं स्मृतं ।
सात्त्विकं राजसं कर्म तामसं त्रिविधं पुनः॥

aneka-janma-sañjātaṁ
prāktanaṁ sañcitaṁ smṛtam
sāttvikaṁ rājasaṁ karma
tāmasaṁ tri-vidhaṁ punaḥ

The accumulated effects of karmas discharged in many past lives is called *sañcita*, it is again subdivided into three: sattvic, rajasic, and tamasic.

(*Devī-bhāgavatam*, 6.10.9)

शुभं वाऽप्यशुभं भूप सञ्चितं बहुकालिकम् ।
अवश्यमेव भोक्तव्यं सुकृतं दुष्कृतं तथा ॥

śubhaṁ vā 'py aśubhaṁ bhūpa
sañcitaṁ bahu-kālikam
avaśyam eva bhoktavyaṁ
sukṛtaṁ duṣkṛtaṁ tathā

Be it auspicious or inauspicious, O King, [the *sañcita-karma*] that is accumulated over a long period must be experienced, be it due to good or bad deeds.

(*Devī-bhāgavatam*, 6.10.10)

जन्मजन्मनि जीवानां सञ्चितानां च कर्मणाम् ।
निःशेषस्तु क्षयो नाभूत्कल्पकोटिशतैरपि ॥

janma-janmani jīvānāṁ
sañcitānāṁ ca karmaṇām
niḥśeṣas tu kṣayo nābhūt
kalpa-koṭi-śatair api

Sañcita-karma, created by the incarnated beings over many previous lives, can never be totally depleted [without being experienced] even in a hundred *koṭi-kalpas* (one hundred million *yugas*).

(*Devī-bhāgavatam*, 6.10.11)

2.2 *Prārabdha-karma* or "actions that have produced fruit"

Prārabdha-karma is the part of *sañcita-karma* destined to directly influence our present life. It is a specific portion of karma extracted from the cosmic bank with which we create our present life. This class of karma is responsible for our current body and conditions. This is ripe karma, ready to be harvested, and therefore, unavoidable.

The same *Devī-bhāgavatam* states the following:

सञ्चितानां पुनर्मध्यात्समाहृत्य कियान्किल ।
देहारंभे च समये कालः प्रेरयतीव तत् ॥

sañcitānāṁ punar madhyāt
samāhṛtya kiyān kila
dehārambhe ca samaye
kālaḥ prerayatīva tat

At the moment of birth, the soul takes a tiny portion of the *sañcita-karma* to come to fruition. It is as if the factor of time induces this process.

(*Devī-bhāgavatam*, 6.10.13)

प्रारब्धंकर्म विज्ञेयं भोगात्तस्य क्षयः स्मृतः ।
प्राणिभिः खलु भोक्तव्यं प्रारब्धं नात्र संशयः ॥

prārabdhaṁ karma vijñeyaṁ
bhogāt tasya kṣayaḥ smṛtaḥ
prāṇibhiḥ khalu bhoktavyaṁ
prārabdhaṁ nātra saṁśayaḥ

This [part of the *sañcita-karma*] is known as *prārabdha-karma* and it gets exhausted only as living beings consume karma. There is no doubt that *prārabdha-karma* must be experienced by living beings.

(*Devī-bhāgavatam*, 6.10.14)

2.3. *Āgāmi-karma* or "present actions"

Āgāmi-karma, also called *kriyamāṇa-karma* or *vartamāna-karma*, are the actions we are currently performing. Part of this karma is transformed into new mental impressions—called *saṁskāras*—that become an integral part of our subtle body. Thus, this karma originates in thought, and through action, it is converted back into thought, because our reactions create new *saṁskāras* as part of this cycle.

In the same scripture, this type of karma is explained in the following way:

क्रियमाणं च यत्कर्म वर्तमानं तदुच्यते ।
देहं प्राप्य शुभं वाऽपि ह्यशुभं वा समाचरेत् ॥

kriyamāṇaṁ ca yat karma
vartamānaṁ tad ucyate
dehaṁ prāpya śubhaṁ vā 'pi
hy aśubhaṁ vā samācaret

> The karma that is being created [by a *jīva*, and that has not yet been completed] is called *vartamāna-karma* (present life karma). After obtaining a body, they [the *jīvas*] execute this auspicious or inauspicious karma.
>
> (*Devī-bhāgavatam*, 6.10.12)

Our present life offers us the wonderful opportunity to settle our cosmic debt. In this life we can burn the portion of reactions, or *āgāmi-karma*, with which we have formed this body and personality, and reduce our *sañcita-karma*. Many, out of ignorance, squander this precious opportunity of human life and instead of reducing their debt, increase it. Instead of diminishing their storehouse of karma, they enlarge it by accumulating new reactions.

If instead of dedicating ourselves to a life of service and religion, we develop new vices, attachments and addictions, new thoughts arise, followed by desires, which lead to actions and ultimately to the creation of more negative karma. Thus, we may die with a greater karmic debt than we were born with.

In fact, the three types of karma comprise what will happen (*sañcita-karma*), what is happening (*prārabdha-karma*), and our reactions to what is happening (*āgāmi-karma*). It is here that we find answers to questions such as free will. Although what is about to happen is inevitable and there is nothing we can do to change what is happening now, we do have the option to freely choose the way we act and respond to what happens.

The *Mahābhārata* says:

हित्वा गुणमयं सर्वं कर्म जन्तुः शुभाशुभम् ।
उभे सत्यानृते हित्वा मुच्यते नात्र संशयः ॥

hitvā guṇa-mayaṁ sarvaṁ
karma jantuḥ śubhāśubham
ubhe satyānṛte hitvā
mucyate nātra saṁśayaḥ

> Abandoning all action, good or bad, developed from qualities, and casting off both truth and falsehood, one becomes emancipated. There is no doubt here.
>
> (*Mahābhārata*, "*Aśva-medha*," 47.11)

Liberation from karma

The mental, emotional, and physical conditions we experience in the present are the result of our previous actions. This chain of cause and effect, of actions and reactions, which keeps us enslaved to the process of repeated birth and death, can easily be cut through with the wisdom of karma yoga. The cycle can be stopped by disidentifying from the process of action and offering the fruit of the works to the transcendental, God, or existence.

The Bhagavad Gita explains this masterfully:

यत्करोषि यदश्नासि यज्जुहोषि ददासि यत् ।
यत्तपस्यसि कौन्तेय तत्कुरुष्व मदर्पणम् ॥

yat karoṣi yad aśnāsi
yaj juhoṣi dadāsi yat
yat tapasyasi kaunteya
tat kuruṣva mad-arpaṇam

Whatever you do, whatever you eat, whatever you offer or give away, and whatever austerity that you perform, do it, O son of Kuntī, as an offering to me.

(Bhagavad Gita, 9.27)

Arjuna thought that if by acting we create the karma that keeps us enslaved to *saṁsāra*, then we should simply stop acting to solve the problem, and so he asked Kṛṣṇa:

अर्जुन उवाच-
ज्यायसी चेत्कर्मणस्ते मता बुद्धिर्जनार्दन।
तत्किं कर्मणि घोरे मां नियोजयसि केशव॥

arjuna uvāca
jyāyasī cet karmaṇas te
matā buddhir janārdana
tat kiṁ karmaṇi ghore māṁ
niyojayasi keśava

> Arjuna said, "O Janārdana! O Keśava, why do you direct me to perform this terrible action if you believe that discernment is superior to action?"
>
> (Bhagavad Gita, 3.1)

What Arjuna is saying, in his argumentative question to Kṛṣṇa, is very significant: if discernment is more elevated than action, then it would be more appropriate either to stop fighting and just sit passively by the roadside, or to accept the renounced order of life, and leave worldly life to live in a cave or forest and do nothing.

However, Kṛṣṇa explains that action cannot be stopped, not even for a moment. It is impossible to escape activity.

न हि कश्चित्क्षणमपि जातु तिष्ठत्यकर्मकृत् ।
कार्यते ह्यवशः कर्म सर्वः प्रकृतिजैर्गुणैः ॥

na hi kaścit kṣaṇam api
jātu tiṣṭhaty akarma-kṛt
kāryate hy avaśaḥ karma
sarvaḥ prakṛti-jair guṇaiḥ

> Everyone is bound to act, helplessly, according to the modes (*guṇas*) of nature (*prakṛti*). Therefore, no one can stop acting, even for a moment.
>
> (Bhagavad Gita, 3.5)

Even if we stop all physical movement, it is absolutely

impossible to stop action completely, since we not only act on the physical level, but on much more subtle levels of the mind and emotions. Even if we stop moving the body, dreams, fantasies, expectations, and imaginations continue to create more karma.

Kṛṣṇa explains that there is a way to act without creating karma: it is not a matter of giving up action, but rather renouncing selfish intentions to obtain results.

त्यक्त्वा कर्मफलासङ्गं नित्यतृप्तो निराश्रयः ।
कर्मण्यभिप्रवृत्तोऽपि नैव किञ्चित्करोति सः ॥

tyaktvā karma-phalāsaṅgaṁ
nitya-tṛpto nirāśrayaḥ
karmaṇy abhipravṛtto 'pi
naiva kiñcit karoti saḥ

> Such people, having given up attachment to the fruits of their actions, are always satisfied and not dependent on external things. Despite engaging in activities, they do not do anything at all.
>
> (Bhagavad Gita, 4.20)

To free ourselves from reactions is to perform actions without ascribing them to ourselves. That is, act without thinking we are the agents or authors of what we do. *Karma-yogīs* directly experience God as the authentic actor, through the three modes of nature or *guṇas*.

A soldier is not responsible for his actions during a

war, as he only performs his duties and executes orders. During his service, he does what his superiors order him to do. If a soldier kills his enemy during a war, he is awarded medals. However, if the same soldier murders his neighbor during peacetime, he is prosecuted for murder and punished by law. Similarly, *karma-yogīs* who act in the service of God and mankind, under the expert guidance of a bona fide spiritual master, are no longer responsible for what they do nor the consequences. In this way, they free themselves from the results of their actions to become a channel through which the stream of life and existence flows.

Karma yoga allows us to understand that we are in fact the ones who adopt the role of doers instead observers. Our mistake is to think we perform, when in reality, our actions happen to us. Karma is created by our attitude to what happens, and if we just observe and do not react, the accumulation of karma stops. *Karma-yogīs* renounce the role of actors to become witnesses, thereby ceasing to take credit for their actions or their actions' results.

We can experience different attitudes when we breathe. If we breathe unconsciously and involuntarily, exhalations will be short and accelerated, reflecting our mental tension. But if we pay attention to the breathing process and accept the role of "actor" or "the one who breathes," we can inhale deeply and exhale by completely emptying the lungs and even hold our breath for a certain period of time. If we accept the position of the witness, which involves just observing without interfering, we can transform this same breathing process from an action that we perform to an event that happens to us. The process of inhaling and exhaling will invite us to dissolve, since without interfering, there is no need for "someone" to breathe.

नैव किञ्चित्करोमीति युक्तो मन्येत तत्त्ववित् ।
पश्यञ्शृण्वन्स्पृशञ्जिघ्रन्नश्नन्गच्छन्स्वपञ्श्वसन्॥
प्रलपन्विसृजन्गृह्णन्नुन्मिषन्निमिषन्नपि ।
इन्द्रियाणीन्द्रियार्थेषु वर्तन्त इति धारयन्॥

naiva kiñcit karomīti
yukto manyeta tattva-vit
paśyañ śṛṇvan spṛśañ jighrann
aśnan gacchan svapañ śvasan

pralapan visṛjsn gṛhṇann
unmiṣan nimiṣann api
indriyāṇīndriyārtheṣu
vartanta iti dhārayan

Let yogis, knowers of Truth, think: 'I do nothing at all.' Even as they occupy themselves with seeing, hearing, touching, smelling, eating, walking, sleeping, breathing, speaking, evacuating, grasping, and opening and closing their eyes, they know that [it is only] the senses [that] operate in relation to their objects.

(Bhagavad Gita, 5.8–9)

When reading this, some people might think that karma yoga can lead to a lack of enthusiasm or even indifference toward our daily obligations. However, observing does not mean adopting a tamasic attitude toward life. What actually happens is exactly the opposite: as we free ourselves from the feelings of obligation, which are always related to others, a deep sense of responsibility will be born within us, which will be directed toward ourselves. Working with the feeling that God is the authentic authority allows us to cultivate a deep and mature inner work ethic. Then, we can act unselfishly, without expectations that blind and hinder us or make us think more about personal benefits and interests than the work itself. Through the art of action, we easily transcend the great obstacle of attractions and aversions on the spiritual path.

There is no specific activity that we can perform that will free us from karma, lead us to bliss, and bring us the happiness that we so long for. Only the wisdom of the Self, like the light of the sun, can extinguish the darkness of ignorance and reveal our authenticity, as Śaṅkarācārya explains very beautifully:

अविरोधितया कर्म नाविद्यां विनिवर्तयेत् ।
विद्याऽविद्यां निहन्त्येव तेजस्तिमिरसङ्घवत् ॥

avirodhitayā karma
nāvidyāṁ vinivartayet
vidyāvidyāṁ nihanty eva
tejas-timira-saṅghavat

> Activity does not have the ability to annihilate ignorance, because it is not in conflict with it. Only wisdom is capable of eliminating ignorance, in the same way that light dispels darkness.
>
> (*Ātma-bodha*, 3)

Meditation in motion is not just observing our actions but observing the very doer. Instead of adopting the position of the "doer," we observe both the action and the "actor." This radical leap from the doer to the witness is a matter of consciousness. The doer is nothing more than a computer with mechanical reactions. Meditation or relaxation guides suggest we stop "doing." It is important to understand that this does not mean ceasing all activity but ceasing to react. The position of a witness requires observation and, therefore, greater awareness. Karma yoga means transforming mechanical reactions into conscious actions, because only through this transformation is it possible to stop the accumulation of karma.

Illusion, or *māyā*, is based on two fundamental mistakes: believing we are the doers and desiring the results of our actions. The mental phenomenon that calls itself "I" claims all activity and sets itself up as the central actor, or the executing center, striving to experience pleasure and escape pain. Illusion is a prison whose bars are the sense of continuity and the illusory stability of the "I." Its chains are claiming authorship for its actions. Its shackles are the search for results through its activities.

Karma yoga encourages us to go beyond selfishness

and transcend the limitations of the small, narrow "I" that lives by taking credit for what happens to it. The consequence of this particular yoga is to open and enlarge the heart, which invites us to become accessible and surrender to transcendental consciousness. As we become possessed by it, our activities cease to be a reflection of illusion, ego, mind, ignorance, and imperfection, and become expressions of light and truth.

An excessively selfish person is incapable of performing a task without thinking of their own benefit. The mind is fixed on the gain that the effort will provide. This wisdom teaches us to act without expecting personal gain of any kind in return for our deeds, as we do when we start a true friendship or when we love someone. Since all goals reside in the future, the search for results prevents us from being present. Pursuing benefits inevitably turns us into "tomorrowists," disconnecting us from the present and pulling us away from the now and, therefore, from reality.

This path teaches us that ambition for mystical attainments is precisely what prevents us from achieving them, for it tenses us and does not allow our action to be meditative. Overcoming the ego and expanding the heart comes to yogis as an indirect and natural consequence, never as a deliberately-pursued result.

In religion, achievements are not the consequence of our efforts. Grace, meditation, devotion, love, peace, truth, enlightenment, and anything elevated are never the product of our techniques, methods, or practices, but only come as an indirect consequence of our way of living.

Karma yoga offers us a way out of the slavery to the *saṁsāra* wheel, showing us another door leading beyond the prison of our mind: a door that leads to awakening to the reality that no one was ever released, because no one was ever imprisoned. No one ever came out because nothing and no one was ever inside.

Abandoning the doer and the results of your works, you will find yourself. Renouncing everything, you will realize that you are only what you cannot give up. Abandon all that you think you possess, all that you consider yours, all that it is possible for you to abandon. Abandon even the renunciation and the person who abandons. That which you are trying so hard to attain is precisely the only thing that is impossible to get rid of.

मुञ्च मुञ्च हि संसारं त्यागं मुञ्च हि सर्वथा ।
त्यागात्यागविषं शुद्धममृतं सहजं ध्रुवम् ॥

muñca muñca hi saṁsāraṁ
tyāgaṁ muñca hi sarvathā
tyāgātyāga-viṣaṁ śuddham
amṛtaṁ sahajaṁ dhruvam

Renounce, renounce the world of appearances; then completely renounce even renunciation. But whether you renounce or not, enjoy the nectar of your natural state. The Self, by its very nature, is immaculate, immortal, and immutable.

(*Avadhūta-gītā*, 3.46)

Only that which you cannot leave is really yours, the only thing that truly belongs to you, your authentic divine nature, what you are. You are what you so greatly desire.

"Acting in the world in accordance with this wisdom, one can aspire to live a hundred years."

Wisdom is required to live in the world without being affected by it. If we have wisdom, we can live for a hundred years and fulfill our duties without them affecting our purity and original freedom. When we love, we feel united with our beloved. When we experience hunger, we identify with the hunger. We do not feel that we experience hunger, but rather that we are hungry. When we feel rage, it completely takes over. If there is fear, we are scared. When we feel sadness, it invades us, permeating every corner of our being. It seems inevitable that our actions, whether physical, mental, or emotional, condition us. Our activity colors us with its tones and leaves its imprint on us. As long as it is executed from the egoic phenomenon, every action affects us.

The only way to act during life without being conditioned by action is to know how to renounce being the doer. To free ourselves from action, we need the wisdom to be witnesses or observers of our actions rather than doers. It is very simple to be the witness because it does not require doing anything, not even thinking. In fact, to stop thinking is the first step to place ourselves in the position of witness to our actions. As long as we continue to think, it will be impossible to place ourselves as witnesses. In order to stop thinking, we must observe thoughts instead of thinking them.

The first thing to discover is that the mind does not belong to you. Society has installed your mind in you through the brainwashing process called *education*. The mind is not part of who you really are, but observation is. As you observe, the domain of the mind loses its power until it becomes irrelevant. This irrelevance of mental activity is the beginning of freedom. To stop being the doer means to stop being the thinker of thoughts, the feeler of emotions, and the doer of activities. Instead, we must take the position of the witness and observe our emotions, thoughts, and activities. Moving from the role of doer to witness requires a radical shift in our lives.

Nowadays, there are many recommendations for thinking, but I advise you to just observe. To analyze or reflect is only to go round and round in a vicious circle. Analysis will take you to the distant past in your memory without giving you a real way out. It will give you a certain degree of understanding about the beginning of your problem, but you will remain the same. You will be able to adjust to the demands of the environment and the parameters of society without any real transformation. Observation, on the other hand, implies a true transformation from the very roots of who you are. It will purify you and remove all conditioning. Although social conditioning has contaminated your roots, your consciousness remains eternally pure, clear, crystalline, and transcendental.

"...without action restricting one's freedom."

By nature, consciousness is freedom; therefore, it does not refer only to what is superficial. You can be free even in a guarded jail cell. Your freedom does not depend on where you are. It is not related to bars or chains, but to consciousness. You can be a prisoner in your own home. You can be a captive in your job. You can be imprisoned in a romantic relationship or a marriage.

It is impossible to be free externally because you are obliged to yield in order to participate in society. You have no choice but to compromise in order to live with peace of mind. If you do not restrain yourself, your freedom will be problematic for others. You have the freedom to listen to loud music at home. However, if it is midnight and your neighbors are sleeping, you will have to limit your freedom. In an interdependent society, our freedom will always be limited. We can live freely as long as our freedom does not limit that of others. In an interdependent universe there is no absolute freedom. Human beings are interdependent, even with the environment.

Absolute freedom is only possible on the level of consciousness. It is achieved through observation without the mind's intervention. Observing, you will realize that you are not greed, anger, jealousy, or inferiority complexes. As you observe your mental activity, you gradually free yourself from labels such as Russian, Peruvian, Chilean, Spanish, or Korean. You steer clear of denominations like Zionist, Capitalist, or Communist. You distance yourself from labels like successful person, loser, or winner. By revealing that you are not the thought, you experience complete freedom from it. Observation leads you to absolute inner freedom. Those who have found freedom in themselves do not look for it on the surface. By finding freedom deep within, you will have no problem accepting external interdependence or even surrendering to it. Remember that capitulating is only for defeated prisoners who have no alternative. Surrender is only for those who have found their freedom.

Mantra 3

असुर्या नाम ते लोका अन्धेन तमसाऽऽवृताः ।
ताꣳस्ते प्रेत्याभिगच्छन्ति ये के चात्महनो जनाः ॥

asuryā nāma te lokā
andhena tamasā''vṛtāḥ
tāṁs te pretyābhigacchanti
ye ke cātma-hano janāḥ

The worlds of demons are covered by blinding darkness. The killers of the soul go to these worlds after death.

COMMENTARY:

"The worlds of demons ..."

Demons are not worthy of anger, hatred, or resentment, but instead, only compassion. Evil beings suffer as much as or more than their victims, since they only externalize their own inner misery. Their actions and behavior are only symptoms of self-destruction.

Do not hate those who try to harm you or hurt you. Believe me when I tell you that demons' destructivity is nothing more than proof of their pain and suffering, for they burn in the same fire they wish to burn others with.

"... are covered by blinding darkness."

Andham tama means "blinding darkness." The Bible says that darkness was the ninth of the ten plagues sent to Egypt.

> וַיֵּט מֹשֶׁה אֶת יָדוֹ עַל הַשָּׁמָיִם וַיְהִי חֹשֶׁךְ אֲפֵלָה בְּכָל אֶרֶץ מִצְרַיִם שְׁלֹשֶׁת יָמִים. לֹא רָאוּ אִישׁ אֶת אָחִיו וְלֹא קָמוּ אִישׁ מִתַּחְתָּיו שְׁלֹשֶׁת יָמִים וּלְכָל בְּנֵי יִשְׂרָאֵל הָיָה אוֹר בְּמוֹשְׁבֹתָם.
> (שמות י', כ"ב-כ"ג)

> And Moses stretched forth his hand toward heaven; and there was a thick darkness in all the land of Egypt three days. They saw not one another, neither rose any from his place for three

days. But all the children of Israel had light in their dwellings.

(Exodus, 10:22–23)

According to *Midrash Tanchuma* (*parashat Bo*), mentioned also by the great medieval Hebrew master Rashi, the ninth plague of darkness lasted six days, not three. For the first three days, the Egyptians were able to move but could not see each other. In the final three days, darkness paralyzed the people to the point that it prevented them from moving and no one was able to move from where they were. The *midrash* mentions two kinds of darkness, according to the opinions of Rabbi Nechemiah and Rabbi Yehuda. The former refers to classic darkness, which originates in the regions of purgatory (*gehinnom*), while the latter comes from the celestial spheres. These masters explain the difference between classic and celestial darkness. The first acts as a curtain that obstructs sunlight. It is the darkness of ignorance that hides the divine presence and drives us to yearn for the light, which is our true nature. As we aspire to Truth, we become aware of this darkness through observation. On the other hand, celestial darkness precedes light. In this darkness, we experience illusory satisfaction. Instead of a lack of light, we experience a false transcendence of light. This darkness is more dangerous because it poses a serious obstacle to our evolutionary development. Remaining in such darkness, with the illusion of having transcended the light, makes us forget our longing for the light.

In describing how darkness affected the Egyptians, the Bible provides us with details about the effect of both types of darkness on humans. During days with classic darkness, "they did not see one another." During the celestial darkness "nor did anyone rise from his place." Each period corresponds to a kind of darkness. For the first three days the Egyptians experienced classic darkness. They felt deprived of light and eager for it. Selfishness blinded them to the point that it was impossible for them to perceive those around them. They yearned for the light, but the darkness prevented them from reaching it. During the second period, they experienced celestial darkness. They became accustomed to the darkness and stopped experiencing it as the absence of light. Because of this, they felt no motivation to even move from where they were. This kind of darkness blocks us.

In addition, the *midrash* highlights the two purposes of the ninth plague. The first purpose was that there were Jews who did not want to leave Egyptian slavery. God ordered the death of those who refused freedom. They were buried in the days of darkness and the Egyptians never knew about this shameful resistance. The esoteric meaning is that the people of Israel embraced the light, while the Egyptians rejected it. The rebels were buried, thus eliminating any vestige of resistance among them. In other words, the path to transcending darkness means removing any vestige of inner resistance and immersing ourselves in the light.

The second purpose was to give the Israelites the opportunity to go through the Egyptians' dwellings unnoticed and identify the valuable objects they had in their chambers. When the light returned, the Israelites asked for donations of valuable objects and the Egyptians could not deny having them, because the Jews already knew exactly where they were located. The esoteric meaning of this purpose is that the Egyptians were trapped in their satisfaction with darkness. It was then that the Jews searched the darkest and most intimate places of the Egyptians and discovered gold and silver. According to the language of Kabbalah, gold and silver represent divine love. By observing into their innermost intimacy, the Jews discovered their love for divinity. Behind these teachings and their profound esoteric meaning, we find an important universal message.

"The killers of the soul..."

At first glance, the expression "killer of the soul" seems a contradiction, because the sacred scriptures teach that the soul is eternal:

अविनाशि तु तद्विद्धि येन सर्वमिदं ततम् ।
विनाशमव्ययस्यास्य न कश्चित्कर्तुमर्हति ॥

avināśi tu tad viddhi
yena sarvam idaṁ tatam
vināśam avyayasyāsya
na kaścit kartum arhati

> That which pervades the entire body, know it to be indestructible. No one can cause the destruction of the imperishable soul.
>
> (Bhagavad Gita, 2.17)

In the same sacred text, we read:

न जायते म्रियते वा कदाचिन्नायं भूत्वा भविता वा न भूयः ।
अजो नित्यः शाश्वतोऽयं पुराणो न हन्यते हन्यमाने शरीरे ॥

na jāyate mriyate vā kadācin
nāyaṁ bhūtvā bhavitā vā na bhūyaḥ
ajo nityaḥ śāśvato 'yaṁ purāṇo
na hanyate hanyamāne śarīre

> The soul is never born, nor does it die. It has not come into being, does not come into being, and will not come into being. It is not slain when the body is slain.
>
> (Bhagavad Gita, 2.20)

A brief explanation is necessary to understand the term *ātma-hana*, or "killer of the soul." Certainly, nothing and no one can kill or assassinate life itself. However, human beings are capable of living as if their souls were dead: suffocating and ignoring them, in other words, murdering them. In this case, the Upanishad refers to those who live in ignorance of their inner reality. This is like suicide because although they do not annihilate the soul, they live as if they were completely devoid of it. Ignoring the soul means overlooking our true nature, or who we really are. We ignore our beliefs about ourselves and focus on others. Our opinions come from our parents, teachers, family, and friends, as well as from society. This is what Rabbi Nachman of Breslov mentions:

> כִּי עַכְשָׁו בַּעֲווֹנוֹתֵינוּ הָרַבִּים חֵן וַחֲשִׁיבוּת הָאֲמִיתִּי שֶׁל יִשְׂרָאֵל
> נָפַל, כִּי עַכְשָׁו עִקַּר הַחֲשִׁיבוּת וְהַחֵן הוּא אֶצְלָם.

> Nowadays, as a result of our many sins, the true grace and importance of the people of Israel have fallen. Now, most of the importance and grace are found with them (others).
>
> (*Likutei Moharan*, *torah aleph*)

In fact, the ego is the product of others; it has been manufactured by society. The serious problem is that our lives are not rooted in reality, but in an idea about who we are that is not authentic, however respectable it may be. The holy Bhagavad Gita refers to the poor unhappy beings who live in complete ignorance of their spiritual dimension:

> तानहं द्विषतः क्रूरान्संसारेषु नराधमान् ।
> क्षिपाम्यजस्रमशुभानासुरीष्वेव योनिषु ॥
> आसुरीं योनिमापन्ना मूढा जन्मनि जन्मनि ।
> मामप्राप्यैव कौन्तेय ततो यान्त्यधमां गतिम् ॥

tān ahaṁ dviṣataḥ krūrān
saṁsāreṣu narādhamān
kṣipāmy ajasram aśubhān
āsurīṣveva yoniṣu

āsurīṁ yonim āpannā
mūḍhā janmani janmani
mām aprāpyaiva kaunteya
tato yanty adhamāṁ gatim

Those cruel and envious beings, who are the lowest of men, are perpetually thrown by me into the ocean of material existence, to various species of demonic life. O son of Kuntī! Repeatedly taking birth amongst the species of demonic life, these people can never reach me. Gradually, they sink to the lowest levels of existence.

(Bhagavad Gita, 16.19–20)

"... go to those worlds after death."

There are several theologies that claim that sinners and demons are condemned to hellfire. But it is very important to understand this issue from the right perspective. Those with dark minds, wherever they are, will no doubt create hellish realities around themselves. Likewise, those with inner beauty will surely project it onto their surroundings and create paradise.

Everyone has their own history. Different families, nations, religions, and traditions create very different minds. Because of these differences, every one generates a world completely different from the world of others. Although we share the same physical location, we live in different places. We may live in paradise while a colleague lives in hell, or vice versa. Our neighbor may live in a heavenly world while we are immersed in the devil's cauldrons.

All human beings inhabit the same planet, but not the same world. We inhabit one planet and inevitably share the same natural world under the same sun. But although the earth unites us, our worlds unfortunately separate us. All dwellers of the planet create the world they live in: exclusive, personal, and private worlds in accordance with individual states of mind. This can be a hell or a paradise, where they unavoidably continue to dwell even after leaving their physical body. Wherever we find ourselves, we continue to project the same world made up of memories, dissatisfactions, fears, doubts, disappointments, insecurities, anxieties, desires, wishes, dreams, and ambitions: a psychological world surrounded by the infinite ocean of unknown existence.

The place we inhabit is physical, but the world we live in is psychological, since it is an emanation of the mind. While we share the same physical world, our psychological world is private. It is a world with an "I" enclosed within great, thick walls of conditioning. The outside world represents the unknown, while the only familiar thing is what we keep within the small space of our personal world. This private world consists of nothing more than a mental accumulation of memories. From time to time, we gather the courage to look beyond the walls, although we immediately return to our private space. Based on the little information we collect, we create images of all things and all people. In our inability to comprehend the vast and unknown ocean, we construct an image of this infinite ocean in our private egoic world and baptize it with names such as God or Brahman. For the most part, these are terms from fuzzy theories and assumptions, not from clear experience.

There are many people who wonder if the mind precedes the world or the other way around, like the chicken and egg causality dilemma. The mind creates the world and, therefore, precedes it. However, the world supports the continuity of mind, which is fundamental. The mind is the cause and the world is the effect, but the world helps perpetuate the mind. They depend on each other. The world is merely a mental projection. However, many novice seekers mistakenly occupy themselves too much with what is projected and less with the source of the projection. It is not the images projected on the screen that are important, but the projector. Those who try to make decorative changes to the reflection will neglect the essentials and confuse religious life for a fierce struggle with the reflection.

Some people are convinced that paradise is a planet or a geographical site that has an actual location somewhere in the universe. They have been promised that when they get there, they will be eternally happy. However, they ignore the fact that the person who goes there is the same person who is here. As Jon Kabat-Zinn says, "wherever you go, there you are." If on earth we are resentful and quarrel with everyone, then in paradise we will fight with the angels and the saints. Even in heaven, we will continue to project our private world. Wherever we go, our mind will follow us. Moving to an *āśram*, a convent, or a yeshiva will not transform us into saints. Nor will our mind abandon us in such locations; it is impossible to escape from ourselves. If you misunderstand this lesson, you will eventually become angry with the *āśram*, monastery, yeshiva, the rabbi, the guru, and perhaps even with God.

Mohandas Karamchand Gandhi (1869–1948), known as Mahātma Gandhi, said: "If you want to change the world, change yourself." He was very right. Human beings have tried just the opposite over many generations through revolutions and wars, which have proven futile. If we do not feel good in our country, we emigrate; if we dislike our city, we move; if we are dissatisfied, we change jobs or romantic partners. However, little by little we transform the new situation into a copy of the previous one. We simply repeat our earlier state because we have changed everything except ourselves. Gandhi was right, because as long as human beings remain the same as they are, there is no possibility of changing their reality and their world. Thus, true inner revolution becomes indispensable.

Many believe that enlightenment means the complete disappearance of the mind, along with the reality it projects. In fact, what disappears is not the mind but its privacy. As it detaches itself from its privacy, it returns to its original state as consciousness. The egoic phenomenon is a privatization that occurs at the level of consciousness. It is impossible to transcend the mind as long as we live in the particular world we have created. Privacy is part of the nature of illusions and fantasies. The mind is the very basis of personality and projects a private world because it is a personal phenomenon. It is impossible to invite our friends to share our dreams at night while we sleep. Reality, on the other hand, always possesses something public; it is related to all things and all beings. It is possible to meet at home, a café, or town square because these places are part of a physical reality that is accessible to anyone who wants to perceive it.

From our earliest childhood, we are trained to be skilled, efficient, and productive. We are programmed to *function*, but we are not educated to *act*. In fact, we do not receive education but programing. We consider ourselves educated, without realizing that we have been programmed. A clock does not act, it functions. A computer carries out certain functions, but it does not carry out actions. Functioning is mechanical; action is conscious. It is surprising that the daily activities of most human beings are more like functions than actions. A robot can be highly skilled and efficient, but never virtuous. No one can be virtuous or kind without conscious actions. If a machine has been programmed to function in a certain way, it cannot be blamed for anything. Only people who have the capacity to commit atrocities can be considered virtuous for their actions.

Confucius said: "Only the virtuous are capable of loving or hating humans." Pride and arrogance usually hide behind goodness and egoic virtue. Efforts to develop a good moral character only feed hypocrisy and arrogance. Instead of cultivating morality, strive to expand consciousness. Virtue is not related to the mind, but to consciousness. Virtue refers to the special beauty of those qualities and actions that have a moral nature. To cultivate virtue, we must live every moment attentive to what is happening around us, present and alert in the now. Being fully aware, our responses to the situations that life presents us will be appropriate. Our actions will be aligned with our physical, mental, sentimental, energetic qualities, and with the totality of life. We will act in complete harmony with everything and everyone. Our actions will cease to be our own and become universal. The whole universe will be present in every word and every movement. We will stop believing that we live our life to allow life to live and express itself through us.

Let's imagine we are walking through the forest on a hot afternoon and we see a flame that could cause a forest fire. Immediately, we grab our canteen and put out the flame. By acting immediately, there is no time left to think. Everything happened so fast that we cannot say that it was something that we did, because we did not have time to think about it. In reality, it was something that occurred in the encounter between the flame, the forest, and the water; we were only a medium. Those of us who have practiced martial arts, or another sport, know that sometimes the actions we perform do not belong to us. This is acting without acting, or allowing life to act through us.

It is said that Prince Huei of Lang watched attentively as the master chef Ting cut an ox. It was impossible to ignore the cook's movements. His knife glided through the meat, cutting gracefully and masterfully yet effortlessly. His back, shoulders, arms, and hands seemed to dance harmoniously. After observing him carefully for a long time, the prince praised the cook's mastery. The cook put the knife aside and replied: "My art consists in forgetting the objects because only the expression of the path through action matters. In my beginnings, when cutting, I used to see only the knife and the meat. Only after three years, I started seeing the ox in its totality. Now, I do not relate only to the objective plane, but it is the spirit that follows the natural contours. The knife penetrates, cuts, and avoids bones and hard flesh effortlessly. An unexperienced cook sharpens the knife monthly. An experienced cook needs to sharpen it once a year. My knife has nineteen years of cutting thousands of oxen without being sharpened. Because it doesn't cut through hard meats or run into bones, it remains new and its blade is as sharp as the first day. My knife does not wear out because it passes only where it is possible to pass. There are always difficult places where I pause to observe and work slowly. At such times, I act very subtly until the meat crumbles of its own accord." The prince said to the master chef: "Thank you very much for having taught me to nurture life, by using it only in what does not consume it."

These are virtuous acts that leave no mark on our inner psychology. Not one of those unresolved actions do we carry into our inner world. Conscious beings respond to every situation that life presents because they live in a constant dialogue with existence. Consequently, they do not have premeditated lists of what to do or not to do, but respond at every opportunity in a unique way according to the specific situation.

Starting in our childhood, we are instilled with a wealth of information. From the very beginning of our lives, we are conditioned by our parents, family, friends, teachers, and preachers. Although the years go by, society changes, and we are no longer the same, this conditioning remains intact. What has been instilled in us remains there, waiting for the right moment to be used. When the appropriate situation arrives, we will react with what was instilled in us in our childhood or adolescence. When faced with the right circumstances, we will react from what we have at our disposal in our memory. How can we expect our reaction to be appropriate to the right context if the situation occurs today but our reaction comes from yesterday? How can we expect our response to be adequate if it comes from twenty years ago but the event occurs now? I do not believe in lists of commandments or codes of conduct that dictate what is permitted and prohibited.

One of the most effective methods of institutionalizing religion has been the creation of law books and codes of conduct. Usually, the most studious followers become experts on the legitimacy of their transgressions. If you do not believe this, look at what happened to the *Shulchan Aruch* in Judaism; clearly I am not referring to the *Kitsur Shulchan Aruch*. Instead of being a guide to inform us about *halachah* (Jewish law), it became the ideal means to find justifications. Many so-called religious people open it to find an appropriate legitimization for a desired transgression. That's why a rabbi *posek* is needed to consult *halachah*.

The manuals of conduct of religious institutions are beneficial for the masses, but not for the individual. For centuries, organized religion has preached that by striving to develop good character, we will enter paradise where we will encounter God. However, this religious preaching is completely wrong. First, people who strive to cultivate good character do not find God. Secondly, the order is reversed because God is found first and then virtue manifests. And only when virtue comes to us naturally, will we enter paradise.

Virtue comes from consciousness and evil comes from unconsciousness. It is impossible to consciously cause suffering to others. If we are conscious of our actions, we cannot purposely harm fellow human beings or lose our minds and become violent. Cruelty can only manifest itself under the shadows of unconsciousness. Evil comes from darkness, blindness, or ignorance. Perversion expresses itself only under the cover of darkness provided by unconsciousness.

Human beings do not need to possess a virtuous or good character, but only to be more conscious. Any character trait, however good, is false. Consciousness is real, true, and authentic, while character is cultivated under a covered consciousness. A kind character is a social necessity that only lets us function better in society. Children are taught companionship, generosity, and support for others in order to have a more peaceful life. Clearly, being good-natured protects against others' egos. It allows us some security because it reduces, to some degree, the possibilities of being hurt. But my path aims for a radical and complete transformation. I do not provide protective elements to make life easier. I do not teach methods to move in the darkness, but to ignite one's own light. This is not a method to cultivate a beautiful character but to awaken. I do not suggest following behavioral norms as dictated by religious organizations. I do not want human beings to live according to a long list of commandments, but to what their consciousness dictates.

Society promotes the cultivation of character since it facilitates the domination of the masses. People with character are easy to control. Since their reactions were previously programmed, they behave more like computers than souls.

People with character are manageable like devices. Their reactions are mechanical. It is possible to know what to say or what to do to elicit certain responses. If we press a certain button, they become exasperated, if we press another, they become uncomfortable, and if we press yet another, they become happy. Programmed responses are not responses, but mere reactions.

It is possible to cultivate the character of a soldier, but not that of an artist. It is possible to cultivate the character of a fanatic, whether communist, rightist, Zionist, or Nazi, but not that of an enlightened being.

Developing a benign and moral character means repressing our negative inclinations. We apply benign character to weaknesses and negative tendencies and suffocate them. But our negative inclinations do not die, they remain repressed within us. Despite acting kindly, someone with character can easily transform into a demon in a moment of weakness. For conscious beings, on the other hand, virtue is only a natural consequence. Their goodness lacks any repression, resistance, or effort because it is part of their nature. People with character are not cheerful, but conflicted. Their character has been developed through inner struggle, rejection, judgment, and self-condemnation. Consequently, they go through life judging and condemning others according to their own moral criteria. They find it very difficult to accept themselves and others.

However, the person of character inspires confidence in the public. It may seem strange to us, but people trust the person of character and feel uncomfortable with an authentic being. Mark Twain said: "Be virtuous and you will be eccentric." A real being inspires fear and insecurity. Many authentic beings have been rejected, imprisoned, tortured, and even killed or crucified throughout history. Only people of moral character tend to pursue careers in politics. But, if we go after consciousness, authenticity, reality, we must prepare ourselves for the opposite reaction by society. In fact, there is no such thing as goodness or evil: consciousness is positive and the absence of it is negative. If we act consciously, our actions will always be appropriate. On the other hand, if we act unconsciously, our behavior will always be inadequate.

Observation, on the other hand, works in the opposite way as character cultivation. By observing our weaknesses, they begin to disappear. Defects are eradicated when illuminated with awareness. Trying to cultivate character, we strive to avoid making the same mistakes. However, in the absence of consciousness, even if we try to change, we will repeat our mistakes. As long as the information we possess about ourselves is nothing more than myths, legends, stories, dreams, and fantasies, change is impossible. Radical transformation is only feasible if we are able to observe our own defects and weaknesses.

Enlightened beings, throughout the ages, have referred to consciousness. On the other hand, priests, pastors, rabbis, imams, and pandits, have preached about the need to cultivate moral character, which is nothing more than a process of conditioning. But the process of awakening does not follow codes of conduct; it only suggests meditation. By being aware of our defects, mistakes, and weaknesses, they disappear. Do not waste your time and energy trying to develop a good moral character. The essential thing is to open your eyes, because awakening is spontaneously followed by morality, virtue, and goodness.

Mantra 4

अनेजदेकं मनसो जवीयो नैनद्देवा आप्नुवन्पूर्वमर्षत् ।
तद्धावतोऽन्यानत्येति तिष्ठत्तस्मिन्नपो मातरिश्वा दधाति ॥

anejad ekaṁ manaso javīyo
nainad devā āpnuvan pūrvam arṣat
tad dhāvato 'nyān atyeti tiṣṭhat
tasminn apo mātariśvā dadhāti

Although the Self is immobile, it is even faster than the mind. The senses cannot reach it because it goes before them. In its stillness, it surpasses the speed of any runner. Mātariśvan maintains the activities of every living being.

Commentary:

From this mantra to the eighth, we witness a brilliant effort to try to describe the indescribable. This effort constitutes a true spiritual treasure for Truth seekers: it is an invaluable direct testimony of transcendental levels that surpass all cultural, religious, and traditional limits.

Anejad ekaṁ

The word *anejat* is formed by *na* and *ejat*. *Ejri* means "to shake" and *na* means "not." The term *anejad* means "stable or motionless." On the other hand, the text says the Self is faster than thought. For a better understanding of the concept of motion, we turn to mechanics, which is the branch of physics that describes the displacement of bodies over time under the influence of specified forces. Motion is a purely physical phenomenon that is defined as an object's change of position in space relative to itself or another object.

Naturally, consciousness is complete and motionless in the tranquility and peace of its own omnipresence. Movement refers to development, change, and transformation in space and time. Consciousness transcends both space and time since it is immutable, fundamental, and essential. Space and time are secondary manifestations that depend on consciousness.

Motion cannot occur without a limited object being absent from a given space. Without spatial limitation, there is no need for motion. It is important to understand that the immobility of consciousness is not restrictive, but is a natural consequence of being omnipresent. It is not that the omnipresent Whole cannot move, but that there is no need for movement because it is already everywhere at once. Perception does not need to move in order to be present in all places and situations.

The term omnipresent combines several Latin elements: the prefix *omni* means "everything," *prae* indicates "before," the verb *esse* means "to be," and the suffix *ente* refers to the present participle. *Omnipresent* is an adjective that describes something that is present everywhere simultaneously. Different monotheistic religions use this adjective to describe divinity, along with omnipotent and omniscient. This has led to historical debates about these capacities in various circumstances. From a non-dual perspective, divine omnipresence exposes the non-existence of the egoic phenomenon. If my existence as something or someone were real, I would be denying divine omnipresence. If I actually existed as an entity, omnipresence would be meaningless. It would be an omnipresence without me, because the absolute would be absent from the space that I occupy.

When read from a mental perspective, the Upanishadic literature abounds in apparent contradictions. The Vedantic view is synonymous with wholeness, while the mind is a partial phenomenon. The mind tries to relate to the world around it from its own fragmentary perspective. It is evident that anything partial has no access to totality; the finite cannot encompass the infinite. From a fragmentary perspective, we perceive conflict and discrepancy. Only from a holistic vision are polarities revealed to be complementary and manifest their coherence, for example, night and day, inhalation and exhalation, man and woman.

The empirical reality of names and forms is a constant change, while observation, or immutable consciousness, remains static. Mistakenly, we consider them to be two phenomena instead of one and the same. Likewise, both the observer and the observed are two interdependent polarities or two perspectives of the same single consciousness.

Brahman is the immutable, infinite, immanent, and transcendent reality. It is consciousness, which is the source of matter, energy, time, space, as well as everything that transcends the universe. In fact, Brahman is the Hindu concept of God. Its nature is described as transpersonal, personal, or impersonal by different schools, as stated in the *Śrīmad-bhāgavatam*:

वदन्ति तत्तत्त्वविदस्तत्त्वं यज्ज्ञानमद्वयम् ।
ब्रह्मेति परमात्मेति भगवानिति शब्द्यते ॥

vadanti tat tattva-vidas
tattvaṁ yaj jñānam advayam
brahmeti paramātmeti
bhagavān iti śabdyate

> The sages who have realized the Absolute, the non-dual knowledge, refer to it as Brahman, Paramātmā or Bhagavān.
>
> (*Śrīmad-bhāgavatam*, 1.2.11)

Enlightenment means realizing that Brahman is the authentic nature and essence of all things and all beings. It means recognizing that the reality is only our experience and not reality itself, since we only experience existence but not consistency. To awaken is to become aware of what we really are.

"Although the Self is immobile, it is even faster than the mind. The senses cannot reach it, because it goes before them..."

The mind and its sensory externalization only become meaningful in the context of the experience of objective phenomena. The mind and the senses become relevant only within the framework of dual and relative experience. They are understood as suitable instruments for functioning within the relative dimension. However, they are useless in the context of subjective reality.

The mind is *ātma-śakti*, the mysterious power of Ātman. It consists of the Self's enigmatic capacity to manifest and express itself. Absolute consciousness expresses itself through the mind as a relative reality of names and forms, that is, as movement. God manifests as the cosmos itself, as relative reality through the mind. In fact, it is the means through which unity appears to be diversity and the One is transformed into many. The mind is the consciousness that identifies with thoughts.

However, no matter how fast you go, wherever you go, you will only find that the omnipresent Self is already there. Wherever we go, however fast we move, we will only find that existence is already present. Wherever we look, we will see that life is always ahead of us. In fact, what we perceive is not the universe, but perception itself. So that no matter how fast we move, wherever we go, we will see that perception is already there. Perception is endearingly subjective; therefore, matter is not inert, but is completely overflowing with vital cognition. Consciousness is what knows the experience, the infinite space where all experience occurs, and the essential substance of all experience. It is its own source and origin, as expressed in the *Vedānta Sūtra*:

अथातो ब्रह्मजिज्ञासा ॥

athāto brahma-jijñāsā

Now, therefore, the inquiry into Brahman.
(*Vedanta Sūtra*, 1.1.1)

And then:

जन्माद्यस्य यतः ॥

janmādy asya yataḥ

> Brahman is that from which everything originates, is sustained, and is dissolved.
>
> (*Vedānta Sūtra*, 1.1.2)

The search for this origin is the search for oneself: for the authentic "I am," which we also read in the Bhagavad Gita:

> अहं सर्वस्य प्रभवो मत्तः सर्वं प्रवर्तते ।
> इति मत्वा भजन्ते मां बुधा भावसमन्विताः ॥

ahaṁ sarvasya prabhavo
mattaḥ sarvaṁ pravartate
iti matvā bhajante māṁ
budhā bhāva-samanvitāḥ

> I am the origin of everything. Everything emanates from me. Having understood me this way, the sages worship me whole-heartedly.
>
> (Bhagavad Gita, 10.8)

The senses are unable to grasp it, not because of remoteness or distance, but because Ātman is the source of them. Likewise, it is impossible to define the Self with words because its existence precedes vocabulary and even thought. The difficulty in understanding the Self through the senses lies in the lack of distance between the subject and its intrinsic reality. The other reason, and perhaps the main one, is that it is impossible to perceive consciousness as an object because it lacks objective attributes. In other words, it is not another object, nor does it belong to objective reality; it is subjectivity itself.

Consciousness consists of an uninterrupted subjectivity that in its constant flow leaves no room for separation or the existence of the "other." Ātman is closer to us than we are to ourselves. Therefore, a quest for it does not involve a sensory apprehension of "something." Its subjective nature demands a much more intimate and endearing cognition more related to "being" than to "knowing." Truth cannot refer to temporal objective experience, therefore it cannot be found through empirical investigation. In order to know it, it should be courted as a true lover.

Inquiring into the nature of consciousness is especially relevant for Advaita Vedanta. It is so important that the third chapter of the *Aitareya Upanishad* dares to call consciousness itself the One without a second or Brahman. It is the only one of the four *mahāvākyas* that suggests Brahman is pure consciousness. It calls it *prajñānam brahma*. *Prajñāna* is consciousness or the very essence of all things and all beings.

Science investigates the empirical or objective world, while spirituality deals with consciousness or subjectivity. While the former investigates the objective dimension, the latter can be considered the science of the subjective. The only difference lies in the direction of the research. In essence, both inquire into the nature of reality. For many years in the West, consciousness was believed to be only a mental expression. The East has always understood that the source of cognitive activity is the non-dual reality of consciousness. Consciousness is characterized not only by knowing every perception or experience, but also knowing that it knows.

Likewise, the essence of both perception and what is perceived is one and the same. To delve deeper into this, it should be clear that everything we know about the universe consists solely of our perception of it. We think we know the universe we inhabit; however, we only know our experience of it. In fact, the only thing we know throughout our lives is perception or experience.

For example, our perception of ourselves, whether on a physical, mental, or emotional level, consists only of a perception of sensations, thoughts, and emotions. We know nothing of ourselves, or of our sensations, thoughts, or feelings. We only know our perception of them. If we analyze our perception, the only substance we will find is consciousness. Consequently, everything that is perceived is composed of perception itself.

Most human beings blindly believe that there is a universe of objects separate from them as subjects. According to this idea, perception is the only relationship between the objective universe and the perceiving subject. It is impossible to locate perception, or consciousness, in a specific physical place, for the simple reason that every physical, mental, or emotional place, as well as every dimension, is nothing but perception. The reality is that perception or consciousness is not located in any particular place, but that all experience takes place within perception. Consciousness is not located in some space or area within our body, but rather we are immersed in consciousness, which is unlocalizable. Perception or consciousness is where all experience takes place.

We believe that there is an "I" that perceives the world through the senses from within a body. However, there cannot be a relationship between this "I" and the universe because they are not two different phenomena. They are one and the same reality. There is no internal entity that perceives an external reality and is disconnected from it. These two supposed elements cannot be related to each other because in perception they are not separated, just as there is no relation between our home and our house or between the ocean and the water. The only substance or raw material of consciousness is perception itself. There is only knowing, perceiving, or experiencing. The illusion, or *māyā*, is believing that there is an inner subject that experiences an outer reality composed of objects. The division between the subjective and objective poles is an illusion because ultimate reality is only the subjectivity of consciousness. Intimate perception is the only thing that exists: a non-dual perception, uninterrupted, and devoid of separate or independent objects.

Mantra 5

तदेजति तन्नैजति तद्दूरे तद्वन्तिके ।
तदन्तरस्य सर्वस्य तदु सर्वस्यास्य बाह्यतः ॥

tad ejati tan naijati
tad dūre tad vantike
tad antar asya sarvasya
tad u sarvasyāsya bāhyataḥ

While moving it is immobile. It is both distant and very close. It is both inside and outside of everything.

Commentary:

In a busy society like ours, we flip through magazines or look at newspapers just to get some information. Unfortunately, there are many who read literature such as the Bible, the Koran, or the Upanishads in the same superficial way. Only a close reading allows us to meditate on the deep truths hidden behind the words.

This verse is a continuation of the previous one. When reading it for the first time, it may seem contradictory and even absurd. *Ejati* means "it moves" and *naijati* means just the opposite, "it does not move." In the Bhagavad Gita, we find the same teaching that this verse shows us:

सर्वेन्द्रियगुणाभासं सर्वेन्द्रियविवर्जितम् ।
असक्तं सर्वभृच्चैव निर्गुणं गुणभोक्तृ च ॥

sarvendriya-guṇābhāsaṁ
sarvendriya-vivarjitam
asaktam sarva-bhṛc caiva
nirguṇam guṇa-bhoktṛ ca

It is inside and outside of all beings; it is mobile and immobile; being subtle, it is incomprehensible, and although it is far away, it is the closest thing.
(Bhagavad Gita, 13.15)

Throughout history, many statements of great sages and prophets have been considered nonsensical or contradictory. Various statements from the Upanishads may seem to be irrational utterances. However, the nuance of an opinion depends on the point of view of the person expressing it. In fact, it is possible to understand different opinions that at first glance seem contradictory. For example, from an egoic perspective, accepting a spiritual teacher is harmful and destructive in many ways. But, on the other hand, if one aspires to significant spiritual development in this life, an enlightened guru can be of great help. Both views are legitimate and even correct, depending on our aspirations.

If we pay attention to the first chapter of the Bhagavad Gita, we will see that several of the arguments made by Arjuna can be easily accepted from an egoic perspective. Likewise, some of Kṛṣṇa's guidance can be rejected by a reader without spiritual aspirations. As Paul says in 1 Corinthians 1:18: "The word of the cross is foolishness to those who perish, but to those who are saved, that is, to us, it is the power of God."

From a relative and dualistic point of view, many teachings of enlightened beings seem nonsensical. For most, the quantum leap from the personal to the universal is madness. In the Hebrew Talmud, insanity, like the innocence of the infant, is thought to be a prerequisite for accessing deeper levels of consciousness.

אָמַר רַבִּי יוֹחָנָן, מִיּוֹם שֶׁחָרַב בֵּית הַמִּקְדָּשׁ נִיטְּלָה נְבוּאָה מִן הַנְּבִיאִים וְנִיתְּנָה לַשּׁוֹטִים וְלַתִּינוֹקוֹת.

(תלמוד בבלי, בבא בתרא, דף י"ב, ע"ב)

Rabbi Yochanan said, "From the day the Temple was destroyed, the prophecy was taken from the prophets and given to fools and babies."

(*Talmud Bavli*, *Bava Batra*, 12b)

אָמַר רַבִּי אַבְדִּימִי דְּמִן חֵיפָה, מִיּוֹם שֶׁחָרַב בֵּית הַמִּקְדָּשׁ נִיטְּלָה נְבוּאָה מִן הַנְּבִיאִים וְנִיתְּנָה לַחֲכָמִים.

(תלמוד בבלי, בבא בתרא, דף י"ב, ע"א)

Rabbi Avdimi from Haifa said: "From the day of the destruction of the Temple, the prophecy was taken away from the prophets and given to the wise ones."

(*Talmud Bavli*, *Bava Batra*, 12a)

Rabbi Moshe Sofer, The Chatam Sofer, explains that there is no contradiction between Rabbi Yochanan and Rabbi Avdimi of Haifa:

וְעַל דֶּרֶךְ זֶה, נִתְּנָה נְבוּאָה לַשּׁוֹטִים, כִּי לִפְעָמִים נִשְׁמַת אָדָם רוֹאָה דְּבָרִים, וְלִבּוֹ אוֹמֵר לוֹ, אֶלָּא שֶׁנִּרְאֶה לוֹ כִּדְבָרִים רְחוֹקִים וְאֵין שִׂכְלוֹ מֵנִיחַ לוֹ לְהוֹצִיא דִּבְרֵי שְׁטוּת כָּאֵלּוּ מִפִּיו וּבֶאֱמֶת הֵם דְּבָרִים נִגְדָּרִים לְמַעְלָה, וּבְעֵינָיו כִּדְבָרִים רְחוֹקִים. וְהַשּׁוֹטֶה, אֲשֶׁר יִרְאֶה- יַגִּיד. כְּגוֹן עֻבְדָּא דְּרַב טַבְיוֹמָא וְכַיּוֹצֵא בָּזֶה.

(חידושי חתם סופר על מסכת בבא בתרא דף י"ב, ע"א)

And in this way (it is said): 'The prophecy was given to fools' for, at times, one's soul sees, and his heart tells him things, but it looks to him like

> weird stuff, and his mind does not let him express such nonsense from his mouth, but in reality these are profound things in the higher (spheres), just in his eyes they seem like weird. But the fool, if he will see these things, will express them. As we saw in the story about Rav Tavyoma.
> (Chatam Sofer, Commentary on *Bava Batra,* 12a)

Both crazy and enlightened people have transcended the frontiers of the mind. There is a great similarity and a great difference between the two. The difference is that whereas insanity is falling from the mental plane, enlightenment is rising above it. Madness is a descent into a dark abyss, while liberation means flying in a clear sky. Both have abandoned the limits of thought; however, the crazy person descends while the enlightened person flies and transcends the plane of ideas.

Language becomes paradoxical as we approach mystery. Today, science faces problems similar to those of mysticism when trying to explain the inexplicable or describe the indescribable, for example, when confronting phenomena such as wave–particle duality. This quantum demonstration empirically proves how numerous particles can typically behave as waves in certain experiments, while they appear as compact and localized particles in others. This dual behavior is typical of objects in quantum mechanics. Particles can exhibit highly localized interactions, while waves exhibit the phenomenon of interference. Stephen Hawking considered wave–particle duality a "concept of quantum mechanics, according to which there is no fundamental difference between particles and waves: particles can behave like waves and vice versa." Such paradoxical statements are worthy of the mysteries of mysticism.

"While moving it is immobile…"

The world is transitory, while consciousness is imperishable. What is apparent constantly mutates, or *vikara*, but what is real transcends change. The world is like a giant spinning wheel. Like the wheel, the superficial reality of names and forms is constantly changing. All that is external has a beginning, middle, and end. Only the central axis, around which the wheel rotates, remains immutable. In our illusion, we live in the constant dynamics of the rim and completely ignore the static center. We constantly move on the dynamic surface without connecting to the peace at the center. Centering ourselves means finding ourselves in the very eye of the hurricane of life.

This verse invites us to accept life in its totality, which means simultaneously allowing for both the rim's movement and center's peaceful stillness. It is not a matter of stopping the movement of the wheel of *saṁsāra*, but of knowing how to place ourselves at the center. To center ourselves is to transcend karma, because nothing ever happens in the central axis.

"It is both distant and very close."

Consciousness is simultaneously the most distant and the most near to us. It withdraws the most when we seek it with the mind and the senses, and we see it as "something." If we think of it as an experience and seek it as such, it becomes inaccessible. This is because consciousness, or perception, is not an experience but is the very essence that knows all experience. Inquiry into consciousness means searching for our own subjectivity. Efforts to solve a subjective problem in the objective dimension only move us away from the solution.

Consciousness is about what is most intimate. It precedes words, emotions, thoughts, and beliefs. It precedes the mind and the senses. Nothing can be closer to us, since it is our true nature. Consciousness is the source and origin of what we believe or think we are; it is closer to us than we are to ourselves. Meditating is approaching ourselves and discovering, paradoxically, the intimacy of the distant.

Perhaps physical terms such as remoteness or closeness are not very appropriate for discussing our inner world. It might be clearer to say that consciousness is intimate or foreign. Because when we seek perception through the senses or the mind, it seems foreign. On the other hand, when we recognize it, we gain access to the intimacy of subjectivity.

Let us never forget that while we may at times feel distant from our source, we are always unified with it.

From the tops of towering trees, the distance between the leaves and the roots seems enormous. But they are always intimately connected, in some mysterious way.

"It is both inside and outside of everything."

The first part of the phrase refers to the immanent aspect of consciousness and the second, to the transcendent. Humans have unlimited potential in the depths of their own beings. But unfortunately, they are unaware this treasure exists. Society educates us to be extroverts and completely neglect our inner selves. There is nothing wrong with living on the outside. However, those who move only on the surface live banal lives. I agree with Anton Chekhov, who wrote: "There is nothing more terrible, insulting, and depressing than banality." As long as one does not observe within, life passes by without any magic.

Meditation is looking within. Living in contact with our inner world does not create conflicts with the mundane; on the contrary, it eliminates them. Meditation transforms our vision and, therefore, by directing our gaze toward the external world we no longer perceive only names and material forms. With the vision that has glimpsed the magic of the inner world, we are able to perceive the Divine in the mundane.

Meditation is about searching within. The recognition of inner consciousness allows us to then recognize it in the world, as the essence of everything and everyone.

This shows us that the outside and the inside are both mental interpretations. They are just directions whose point of reference is the idea of the "I," in other words, the egoic conception is the foundation for both the "inside" and the "outside." The point of reference of both is the idea of the "I." Without the walls of the room, there would be no concepts such as inside or outside. If the walls collapsed, the notion of inside or outside would disappear. Truth is both immanent and transcendent; it lies both inside and outside of everything and everyone; it resides in the individual and the universal.

The term *exterior* refers to the objective world of names and forms. The term *interior* refers to subjective reality. Going after our inner self means detaching ourselves from the objective in order to perceive our perception. Undoubtedly, this verse elevates us above the well-known debates between believers and atheists about the existence of God. The verse definitively tells us that outside of God nothing exists and that the only reality is God.

In fact, it is impossible to divide experience into parts that are closer or farther. Experience does not allow for divisions of any kind. The sound of an airplane is no more distant than my thoughts. That mountain I see is no farther than the palm of my hand. Actually, all we know of the sound of the airplane's engine is what we hear. All we know about the mountain is what we see. This is also the case for my thoughts or the palm of my hand. Hearing, seeing, smelling, and touching happen here. But I am not referring to a "here" that indicates a physical place located in space, but to an unlocalizable subjectivity. "Here" is a subjectivity that fills the totality of experience.

Consciousness is generally believed to be something that lies within us. Likewise, we believe the objective universe resides beyond our senses as something completely separate from who we are. In reality, we are not on a planet, instead, all the galaxies and stars are within us. We are not located anywhere, for all places are found within what we are. Everything and everyone is within this endearing subjectivity. In my childhood, I loved to look at the stars and enjoy their beauty and their mysterious silence, which hides a thousand secrets. At night, we can see the constellations twinkling in the supposed distance. However, the only thing we know about them is the experience derived from our observation. Such observation occurs in the "here," within the intimate subjectivity of our own being. In the experience of observation, there is neither space nor distance.

The mind divides the subjectivity of perception into a "someone" and a "something." As it interprets, the mind fragments the experience into two apparent phenomena: a subject that perceives an object through its senses. The subject is the observer and the object is the observed. However, such apparent fractioning takes place only at the level of thought; therefore, it is theoretical and not factual in nature. Beyond all the worlds created by thought and its interpretations, the only thing that exists for consciousness is the indivisible and uninterrupted subjectivity of itself.

When we close our eyes, our experience of the universe become no more than the song of a bird, the ticking of the clock, and the contact between our back and the armchair. According to the mental interpretation of such an experience, these three objects are separate elements, that is, objects, while I am the subject. Consistent with the information provided by our mental interpretation, the bird's twittering comes from a feathered vertebrate singing at a certain distance from me. Likewise, the armchair is composed of inert matter, whose sensation I perceive on my back, very close to me. However, our mental interpretation differs radically from direct experience. To clearly appreciate the difference between the two, we must observe the experience attentively without mental intervention, which would be equivalent to observing without interpretation. This is what meditation is all about, observing without the intervention of thought. The ego is nothing more than the mental interpretation we have developed about what we are. Therefore, an observation without the participation of thought means observing the world free of any perspective or point of view, or if you prefer, observing reality from the perspective of a newborn child. I am referring to that refreshing vision that Pablo Neruda sought so much and that I see reflected in his poem *Al pie desde su niño* (At the foot of his child):

A child's foot doesn't know it's a foot yet
And it wants to be a butterfly or an apple
But then the rocks and pieces of glass,
the streets, the stairways
and the roads of hard earth
keep teaching the foot that it can't fly,
that it can't be a round fruit on a branch.
Then the child's foot
was defeated, it fell
in battle,
it was a prisoner,
condemned to life in a shoe.

Direct experience is like the foot of a child who does not yet know that it is a foot. It is like looking at the world as if it were our first moment on the planet. It is like experiencing the world without knowing what birds, backs, or armchairs are. Free from the ideas of birds, backs, or armchairs, we do not think of them as objects different from the experience of listening or perceiving. In the absence of interpretation, the bird's song is one with us as conscious presence. The experience of hearing is non-dual in nature; therefore, it is not divided between a listener and the experience of listening. The recognition of non-dual reality is called *yoga*.

योगश्चित्तवृत्तिनिरोधः ॥

yogaś-citta-vṛtti-nirodhaḥ

> Yoga is the cessation of all mental activity.
>
> (*Yoga Sūtra*, 1.2)

According to Patañjali Maharṣi, *yoga*, or "union," is a state devoid of mental activity. It is therefore an observation free of all mental interpretation, both of the world and of ourselves.

Both the experience of listening and the conscious presence that we interpret as the listener "I" share an identical and unique substance. Just as the ocean and the waves are water, consciousness is the authentic essential nature of both the experience and the experiencer. There is no substantial difference between the conscious presence, or subject, and the experience of listening. The substance of both is perception; it is the same subjective and endearing awareness.

Let us return to the armchair. When we close our eyes and remove the visual image of the object, our experience of the armchair is limited to our sensation of touch; that is to say, our experience of the armchair in its totality is constituted by the sensation of contact with our back resting against it. The armchair's reality does not accept the fragmentation between perceiving subject and perceived object.

Experience as such does not recognize in itself anything as inert or dead, rather it perceives itself charged and overflowing vital cognition or "beingness." If we turn to our mental interpretation of experience, our conclusion will be radically different from that of perception. Although it is true that we perceive, the perceived object is nothing more than a conjecture or supposition. Accepting such an interpretation means neglecting and ignoring the fact that the vision of the armchair, substantially and qualitatively speaking, consists of nothing more than the experience of seeing.

The inwardness and subjectivity of the Self is all that really exists. Only the mind and its illusory inferences appear to fragment this uninterrupted subjectivity. In mental deductions, a division of endearing subjectivity into "I" and "not-I" takes place. The supposed existence a dual phenomenon is meaningless in the context of experiential reality; its existence is relevant only from the point of view of thought. It is important to clearly understand that there are two worlds: the theoretical and the factual. The former is the world formed by ideas, conclusions, concepts, assumptions, suppositions, conjectures, hypotheses, and beliefs. The factual world, on the other hand, is the reality of direct, unmediated experience.

The phrase "rubbing your palms together" contains a certain idea and imagination: this is the theoretical world. Now, rub your hands together without saying a word and pay attention to the sensation. This experience belongs to the factual world, devoid of mental interpretation. The problem with human beings is that they move from and within a theoretical reality, a dream, a fantasy. Their ignorance lies in the fact that they lack access to factual reality and live in complete ignorance of it. Even in the scientific domain, humanity conducts experiments, but often on theoretical grounds. The world is not as the vast majority of human beings experience it. We must wake up to the simple fact that no one reads these lines and no one writes them, everything that happens consists of an accumulation of sensations, interpreted as our "I."

Let us continue our discussion by paying attention to the body, which is an essential aspect of what we apparently are or suppose ourselves to be. We think we are beautiful or ugly, fat or skinny, tall or short. We believe we know what our physical body is and it is ours. However, if we look at it carefully, we will find that the only real and true knowledge we possess about our head, arms, legs, shoulders, and back, as well as the totality of our body, are the many sensations we experience. A mental drawing of our physical morphology gives us an idea about the limbs of our body. However, for direct experience, our body is only an accumulation of sensations.

For example, we all agree that our head is a sphere on a torso, that it is situated between our shoulders and that it has eyes, a mouth, a nose, ears, and a forehead. However, by focusing solely on our sensations, we will discover that our head is something entirely different. Rather than being a sphere between our shoulders, it appears to be a hole in the middle of the universe, a great void through which perception flows continuously. A mental interpretation suggests that the physical sensations are very close while the stars are at a great distance. However, according to direct factual experience, both experiences are equally subjective. Both are of the same intimate nature, that is, they are substantially one and the same with conscious presence.

Many believe they know what the mind is. There are those who teach methods to control it and techniques to develop it. Many books have recently appeared about the mind and how to calm or pacify it. However, the only thing we really know about the mind is the experience of thinking. There is no substantial distance or difference between us, as a conscious presence, and the experience of thought; we are intimately one and the same. In popular belief, the "I" is a separate entity and the closest things to the "I" are feelings and thoughts. We believe that our mental and emotional activity is located in the intimacy of our inner world. In our interpretation, we place the boundaries of our inner world, or what we consider "I," at the skin of our physical body. The skin is supposedly be the most distant thing from us, yet still an integral part of who we believe ourselves to be.

In our mental interpretations, the objective universe is something completely separate from us. We think that this reality made of names and forms consists of something entirely different from what we think we are. We believe we know something about the universe; however, it is nothing more than the experience of perceiving. We believe that the experience of tasting or smelling is more distant from our "I" than our experience of thinking or feeling. Yet all of this is inseparably one and the same with who we are. As the *Chāndogya Upanishad* states:

सर्वं खल्विदं ब्रह्म ।

sarvaṁ khalvidaṁ brahma

All of this is truly Brahman.

(*Chāndogya Upanishad*, 3.14.1a)

Our interpretation of reality presumes the existence of two different phenomena: one as "I" and the other as the experience of perceiving. However, the reality is that there is only the indivisible intimate subjectivity of experience. Whatever exists, for it will be constituted by experience, which in turn is only the intimate subjectivity of our beingness. Our mental interpretation makes us believe that we know objects, but our experience tells us that we only know our experience of them, or, to be more exact, we only know experience. Its non-dual nature does not accept that it can be known by anything or anyone other than itself; therefore, only experience knows itself. Awakening to ultimate reality means realizing that there is only consciousness experiencing itself.

MANTRA 6

यस्तु सर्वाणि भूतान्यात्मन्येवानुपश्यति ।
सर्वभूतेषु चात्मानं ततो न विजुगुप्सते ॥

yas tu sarvāṇi bhūtāny
ātmany evānupaśyati
sarva-bhūteṣu cātmānaṁ
tato na vijugupsate

One who sees everything and everyone in the Self alone, and sees the Self in everything and everyone, does not hate anything or anyone.

COMMENTARY:

The human mind is an island of slavery in the infinite ocean that is a life full of alternatives. In an eternal and infinite existence, rich in possibilities, the chains of mental conditioning reduce our movement to a single direction. We do not move around the world pursuing anything or anyone but fleeing from everything. So, we should not be surprised that at the end of our journey we find ourselves empty-handed. Many people claim to be searching for something in their lives. The truth is that we confuse fleeing from suffering with searching for happiness. We think we are looking for love, but in fact we are trying to elude loneliness. We claim to aspire to freedom, but what we are really doing is running away from oppression. We believe we seek wealth, but in fact we only fear poverty. We think we take care of ourselves, but in reality, we are hypochondriacs who escape illness. We think we seek paradise, but we only aspire to avoid hellfire. Instead of going after something, humanity lives in constant flight. The energy that fuels our ambitions comes from fear, not inspiration.

Although we think we aspire to feelings of shelter, safety, and security, in reality we only run away from unpleasant and uncomfortable experiences. We try to escape by evading limitation, belittlement, insecurity, loneliness, and pain. What we endlessly seek is refuge from shame, disappointment, sadness, boredom, and conflict. We try to diminish our distress, frustration, misery, and suffering.

Although we believe we are pursuing bliss, in fact we only seek relief and comfort. In this way, we confuse temporary painkillers with the happiness we long for. But instead of granting us bliss, such sedatives transform us into slaves of multiple addictions.

Our entertainment-focused culture only provides us with temporary palliatives. Bliss does not lie in feeling less anguish, nor silence in hearing less noise. Just as freedom is not the absence of slavery, happiness is not the absence of suffering. If we focus on freedom from tyranny, we may one day succeed in reaching a state devoid of oppression, but not in achieving freedom. Being free means much more than not being a slave. Freedom from a certain phenomenon is not genuine, but only a reaction to that phenomenon, and consequently, a continuation of it. This movement, called *dveṣa* or "rejection" in Vedanta, can only lead us to frustration. Emancipation from oppression does not lead to absolute love, freedom, and bliss. Those who escape from reality do not gain access to Truth, because they strive for a solution to their problems instead of seeking awakening.

Most spiritual methods offer solutions in the form of techniques. However, Truth cannot be reached with a technique, because we are the problem. We do not have a problem nor are we its victims, but we are the problem. We are discussing a subjective problem, and therefore, objective solutions are ineffective. Solutions can be applied to the objective plane, but this problem is subjective. It is impossible to defend ourselves from a tiger in our dream with a weapon we left on the bedside table. To protect ourselves from a dream creature, we require a weapon that is effective within the realm of our dream experience. In a similar way, subjective problems can never be resolved with objective solutions.

No activity or practice within the film, no matter how spiritual, will cause one of the characters to pay attention to the screen. Regardless of the effectiveness of the solution, the result of any technique will be the same problem disguised with a supposed solution. Solutions are mechanical, while the real difficulties of life are organic. The real problem is the mind and not the troubles it creates and then tries to resolve. Until we understand this, we will continue to look for techniques and methods to provide us with solutions.

The mind is only capable of facing problems from within its own conditioning. Therefore, its solutions are born from its conditioning and will only aggravate problems. The mind can never find a solution because it is part of the problem. It is impossible for a limited mind to transcend its own limitations. Therefore, my advice is to stop the quest for solutions and simply observe. Although observation is not a solution to inconveniences, it can show us how illusory they are. I am not referring to objective inconveniences, but life's subjective complications. Obviously, observation is not very useful for technical inconveniences such as repairing a cellphone, television, automobile, or computer. But it is useful for subjective and emotional difficulties such as jealousy, envy, resentment, loneliness, and personality complexes.

The real difficulty of human beings is subjective in nature. Their great problem is ignorance, even of the problem itself. Observation does not *resolve* problems; it *dissolves* them. Most of our troubles come from lack of observation and unconsciousness. This process is much simpler than eliminating the problem through a solution. What I am referring to is the dissolution of the problem at the very moment it is observed. All problems originate from and are based on blindness. If the problems are caused by blindness, they can obviously be eliminated by sight. When we observe carefully, we see that problems are born, they overtake us, and dominate our life. They blind us to the point that we begin to sleepwalk. Observation, on the other hand, is like a powerful acid that completely dissolves the essence of the problem.

In our origins, we are divine consciousness, omniscient and omnipresent. However, when we identify with a form, we perceive ourselves to be limited and incomplete. Because of this misperception, we live with a deep sense of lacking something that continually motivates us to complete ourselves. We waste our lives working in exchange for money to acquire and accumulate all kinds of objects with the aim of completing ourselves. We also look for people to complete us. However, no matter how much we hoard objects and people, we continue to experience the feeling of lacking something. The reality is that nothing and no one can complete us, because as consciousness, we are already plenitude itself. The realization of consciousness as our authentic nature means absolute peace and bliss. In Hebrew, the word for 'complete' is *shalem*, which comes from the same grammatical root as *shalom*, or "peace." This implies that genuine peace manifests itself only in those who have realized that they are complete. This experience is born with the awakening to the reality that since we are the One without a second, we are and always have been plenitude itself. In reality, we not lacking anything at all.

"One who sees everything and everyone in the Self alone."

According to this phrase, nothing belongs to us. Everything, including ourself, is only Ātman, or "consciousness." We are neither the owners of anything nor the masters of anyone. Likewise, everything that we like or dislike is just consciousness.

There are those who mistakenly think that spiritual life means having contempt for the world. They think that to become a spiritual person, they should despise this world and aspire to the afterlife. They incorrectly conclude that seeking something spiritual requires hating everything material. They are supposedly religious people whose so-called spiritual aspirations are expressed in the form of hatred of everything related to this world. They think that rejecting the world is a sign of holiness, but holiness can only be born of an inclusive attitude that identifies a single nature as the essence of everything and everyone.

Enlightenment does not allow anyone or anything to be excluded because it is the profound realization that all things and beings are divine in essence. The path of the soul points toward the expansion of consciousness. If in the beginning we love our country and our family, when we advance, we will not reject them, but will love all the countries and families of the world. Most human beings consider the universe, with all its objects, galaxies, planets, plants, animals, human beings, and so on, to be an external phenomenon far removed from themselves. They perceive the existence of the universe as separate from their individuality. On the contrary, Upanishadic wisdom points out that the same essence resides behind the names and the forms that constitute what we perceive as the world. All forms appear within the confines of the one consciousness. Nothing exists outside such perception. Awakening to consciousness brings with it the realization that everything resides in our being or that we are all that is. The Mosaic tradition, through the Torah, illuminates this point as follows:

> לֹא תִקֹּם וְלֹא תִטֹּר אֶת בְּנֵי עַמֶּךָ וְאָהַבְתָּ לְרֵעֲךָ כָּמוֹךָ אֲנִי ה'.
> (ויקרא י"ט, י"ח)

> You shall not take vengeance or bear a grudge against your people. Love your neighbor as yourself. I am the Lord.
>
> (Leviticus, 19:18)

Since we are manifestations of a single consciousness, our neighbor is not a phenomenon different from us. Jesus referred to the above verse and said, "Thou shalt love the Lord thy God with all thy heart, and with all thy soul, and with all thy strength" (Deuteronomy 6:5), and "on these two commandments, hang all the law and the prophets" (Matthew, 22:40). These commandments instruct us to love God and our neighbor as we love ourselves. The deeper meaning is that there is only one nature that resides in our neighbor as well as in us. It is love, which we call God.

Jīvan-muktas, or those "liberated in life," are not conditioned by *rāga* and *dveṣa*: attachments and aversions do not dominate them. They are free of attachment and hatred. Their vision is integral because they see everything and everyone as parts of themselves. For a sleepwalking society, these truths are difficult to accept and impossible to digest.

Vedanta is a process with several steps that lead to become *viśvātman,* or "the *ātman* of the universe." The initial stage is the bodily aspect in which consciousness is confined to physical limits. At the elementary level, we are only concerned with the well-being of our physical form. At this instinctive and animal level, happiness is confused with sensory enjoyment. Next come human beings, who are concerned with the well-being of their loved ones and devote themselves to the welfare of their family and others to whom they have become attached. This category includes those who put the happiness of their partner and children before their own. Next comes the level of consciousness, which includes concern for the environment and the inhabitants of our neighborhood or our city. Higher still are those who embrace the needs of their fellow citizens, of their country, town, or nation. Those who reach this level work and strive, with an altruistic spirit, for the society in which they live. One step higher are the human beings who work for humanity as a whole. In this area, we find all kinds of activists and philanthropists.

However, *viśvātmans* perceive human society as only a small portion of the universe. Their actions aspire to the welfare of the entire universe, since from their perspective it consists of a homogeneous unity. All things and all beings that exist in the universe are parts of an indivisible unity.

By perceiving ourselves as forms or objects located within a specific body, we think the universe is a diversity of objects external to our own reality; it is as if the boundaries between the inner and the outer were demarcated by our skin. Our existence as individuals is an integral part of the universe. This mantra describes a basic characteristic of the perspective of awakening to the reality: essentially, we are the Self. For one who perceives what is, as it is, everything manifests within the field of the one indivisible consciousness. Although we may consider ourselves insignificant in the vast universe, nothing and no one is disconnected from the one Self. As an integral part of our body, even the tip of our pinky finger is relevant. Repulsion, rejection, and hatred vanish when we perceive our individual existence as an integral part of the universe. Only then do we awaken to unconditional love and perceive the love that life embraces us with.

The Bhagavad Gita points this out:

अनन्याश्चिन्तयन्तो मां ये जनाः पर्युपासते ।
तेषां नित्याभियुक्तानां योगक्षेमं वहाम्यहम् ॥

ananyāś cintayanto māṁ
ye janāḥ paryupāsate
teṣāṁ nityābhiyuktānāṁ
yoga-kṣemaṁ vahāmy aham

But to those who always worship me with exclusive devotion, meditating on my transcendental form – to them I give what they lack and I preserve what they have.

(Bhagavad Gita, 9.22)

In perceiving perception or being conscious of consciousness, the entire universe is perceived as an inner or subjective phenomenon. The world is understood as inseparable from our innermost reality. The revelation that the universe is part of our inner world leads to realize our absolute oneness with the Whole.

ममैवांशो जीवलोके जीवभूतः सनातनः ।
मनःषष्ठानीन्द्रियाणि प्रकृतिस्थानि कर्षति ॥

mamaivāṁśo jīva-loke
jīva-bhūtaḥ sanātanaḥ
manaḥ-ṣaṣṭhānīndriyāṇi
prakṛti-sthāni karṣati

An eternal portion of myself, having become an individual embodied soul in this world, associates with the senses, including the mind, and activates them.

(Bhagavad Gita, 15.7)

This verse alludes to the essence of who we are, an eternal portion of divinity. God resides in us as our innermost nature. Our true nature is divine.

This is the final conclusion of Upanishadic literature. The *Bṛhad-āraṇyaka Upanishad* (2.5.19) says: *ayam ātmā brahma* or "This Ātman is Brahman." And, and in the same Upanishad we find the very famous phrase: *ahaṁ brahmāsmi* or "I am Brahman" (1.4.10).

In the *Chāndogya Upanishad* (6.8.7), in the dialogue between Uddālaka and his son Śvetaketu, we also find the great *mahā-vākya*: *tat tvam asi* or "You are That," which indicates that our very essence is "That," which is beyond all verbalization because it constitutes the very origin of words. The great Ādi Śaṅkarācārya expresses it masterfully in his famous formulation *brahma satyaṁ jagan mithyā jīvo brahmaiva nāparaḥ*, or "Brahman is reality, the world is false, and every *jīva* or individual is Brahman."

When the bubble bursts, it discovers that it is actually just water. Similarly, the ego reveals itself to be an infinite space of pure consciousness when it releases the air it seems to enclose.

Undoubtedly, one of the most exciting moments described in the Torah is the creation of human beings.

> וַיִּיצֶר ה' אֱלֹקִים אֶת הָאָדָם עָפָר מִן הָאֲדָמָה וַיִּפַּח בְּאַפָּיו נִשְׁמַת חַיִּים וַיְהִי הָאָדָם לְנֶפֶשׁ חַיָּה.
> (בראשית ב', ז')
>
> Then the Lord God formed man (*Adam*) of the dust of the ground (*Adamah*) and blew into his nostrils the breath of life; and man became a living soul.
>
> (Genesis, 2:7)

Man was not a living being before God breathed His breath of life into him. The *Zohar* tells us that "he who breathed, breathed from his depths," so we understand that what we really are is divinity. God breathed his own breath of life into Adam, so it is nothing less than divinity that is deep within us or the essence of who we are.

"... does not hate anything or anyone."

Many people, even some so-called masters, incorrectly

consider hatred to be the opposite of love. Hatred is actually the opposite of attachment, which is in fact hatred in disguise. Love is about offering, giving, and serving without expectations, while attachment is a type of addiction and need. Although both are similar, attachment is a business that engages us only to the extent that we feel rewarded and receive what we desire. However, when we lose all hope of reciprocation, attachment transforms into hatred. Attachment to people leads to conflict because whoever we are attached to becomes a means to our ends, and no one likes to be used in this way. In the end, with the same vehemence with which we expressed appreciation, hatred can eventually manifest in us. Like a pendulum, our current hatred is usually proportional to our earlier attachment.

Without mentioning it, this text gives us guidance for love. The world's conflicts are rooted in hatred. Hatred persists because no one has tried to teach it, but love has been destroyed because society has been trying to teach us to love for many generations. Whether through politics, the educational system, or institutionalized religion, we have been commanded to love our parents, our enemies, the flag, or religious authorities, to such an extent that love has been stripped of all authenticity.

Our capacity to love is the worst enemy of law and order. Society needs controlled and obedient individuals, but when we love, we lose control of our lives and do not mind acting against social conventions. Society fears the real nature of human beings in their natural and innocent state. We do not possess love; we are possessed by it. And there is no law or authority that can stop a heart overtaken by true love.

Although it only mentions hatred, this mantra leads us to love. It does not tell us that enlightened sages "love everything and everyone," because hate hides love. The absence of hate allows for the natural and spontaneous flow of love. Whoever does not hate anything or anyone, in reality only loves. Hatred is the only reason that love does not shine in its full splendor. Our efforts must be directed toward purifying ourselves of hatred. This is the only way is to awaken to the reality that all things and all beings exist within us. Love cannot be created because it is already the eternal and absolute essence of life. But it is possible to get rid of hatred, in a process similar to cleaning a dust-covered mirror, as Śrī Caitanya Mahāprabhu expresses in the first verse of *Śikṣāṣṭakam*:

चेतोदर्पणमार्जणं भवमहादावाग्निनिर्वापणं ।

ceto-darpaṇa-mārjaṇaṁ bhava-mahā-dāvāgni-nirvāpaṇaṁ

> Glory to the chanting of the holy name of Lord Kṛṣṇa, which cleanses the heart of all the dust, accumulated for years, and extinguishes the fire of conditional life, of repeated birth and death.

There is no need to acquire a mirror because we have one within us. By wiping away the dust that covers it, the mirror will be unveiled. Similarly, we only need to purify ourselves of the accumulated hatred that hides love. Hatred is not a lack of love, but exacerbated selfishness that makes us see others as a means to satisfy our desires and inclinations. We feel attachment for everything that can serve our interests and, on the contrary, we hate whatever prevents us from satisfying our desires. One who awakens to the reality that all that exists is God no longer hates anything or anyone, just as Lord Kṛṣṇa explains to the warrior Arjuna:

सर्वभूतस्थमात्मानं सर्वभूतानि चात्मनि ।
ईक्षते योगयुक्तात्मा सर्वत्र समदर्शनः ॥
यो मां पश्यति सर्वत्र सर्वं च मयि पश्यति ।
तस्याहं न प्रणश्यामि स च मे न प्रणश्यति ॥

sarva-bhūta-stham ātmānaṁ
sarva-bhūtāni cātmani
īkṣate yoga-yuktātmā
sarvatra sama-darśanaḥ

yo māṁ paśyati sarvatra
sarvaṁ ca mayi paśyati
tasyāhaṁ na praṇaśyāmi
sa ca me na praṇaśyati

Harmonized by yoga, the sage sees that the Self resides in all beings, and all beings in the Self; he sees the same in everything and everyone. He

who sees me in everything and everything in me
never parts from me and I never part from him.
(Bhagavad Gita, 6.29–30)

When the light of universal vision shines, the darkness of hatred fades away, revealing unconditional love.

Mantra 7

यस्मिन्सर्वाणि भूतान्यात्मैवाभूद्विजानतः ।
तत्र को मोहः कः शोक एकत्वमनुपश्यतः ॥

yasmin sarvāṇi bhūtāny
ātmaivābhūd vijānataḥ
tatra ko mohaḥ kaḥ śoka
ekatvam anupaśyataḥ

What can cause suffering or illusion to the enlightened ones, those who have realized that all things and all beings are their own self, and who only perceive unity wherever they look?

COMMENTARY:

The previous mantra states that the natural consequence of enlightenment is the absence of hatred. It explains that awakened beings do not experience aversion toward anything or anyone in this world. The current mantra expounds the same but from a positive point of view: they do not hate because they perceive the unity of all things and all beings. *Jīvan-muktas*, or those "liberated in life," are free from the reactions of rejection that are common to the ordinary mind, for they know that they share the same essence with all things and all beings.

"To the enlightened ones, those who have realized that all things and all beings are their own self ..."

If you hug someone, you never think that this is an action performed only by your upper limbs. When you run, it is not only your legs that run. It is not your hand that turns on the stove. All these are considered our activities. No one perceives their own organs as if they were completely different from themselves. In the ordinary state of consciousness, our experience is that we are the ones who hug, run, breathe, or drink because we think of the body and its limbs as manifestations the same person. We recognize that behind the different parts of the body and their various functions, there is a single being and with the different body parts that act as a harmonious unit. Even though ice cream touches your mouth, you are the one who enjoys it. Even if the knee is injured, you feel the pain. By recognizing that your hands, mouth, tongue, legs, and knees are directly connected to you, the attention is focused on you.

In our empirical experience of the dual dimension of names and forms, we perceive a diversity of separate entities. However, in the state of transcendental consciousness, or enlightenment, the experience is that each and every one of us is a member of the same body, which is the manifestation of the Self or God. Beyond the apparent diversity, we center ourselves in the Self or the core of existence. All branches of yoga suggest practices to create the situation conducive to awakening to the Self as the center and origin of all that is. As the Bhagavad Gita confirms:

अहं सर्वस्य प्रभवो मत्तः सर्वं प्रवर्तते ।
इति मत्वा भजन्ते मां बुधा भावसमन्विताः ॥

aham̐ sarvasya prabhavo
mattaḥ sarvam̐ pravartate
iti matvā bhajante mām
budhā bhāva-samanvitāḥ

I am the source of all creation. Everything emanates from me. The sages who know this worship me lovingly with all their hearts.

(Bhagavad Gita, 10.8)

True religion is not about mere rites and ceremonies; it is not simply about particular dress codes or long lists of prohibitions; it is not just about talking, discussing, and evaluating what happened to some extraordinary beings in the distant past. This mantra presents the same Upanishadic vision that Lord Kṛṣṇa transmits to us:

समं सर्वेषु भूतेषु तिष्ठन्तं परमेश्वरम् ।
विनश्यत्स्वविनश्यन्तं यः पश्यति स पश्यति ॥

samaṁ sarveṣu bhūteṣu
tiṣṭhantaṁ parameśvaram
vinaśyatsvavinaśyantaṁ
yaḥ paśyati sa paśyati

The supreme Lord dwells equally in all beings and the imperishable is within the perishable. One who sees in this way, actually sees.
(Bhagavad Gita, 13.28)

This is also confirmed by the *Kena Upanishad*:

भूतेषु भूतेषु विचित्य धीराः ।
प्रेत्यास्माल्लोकादमृता भवन्ति ॥

bhūteṣu bhūteṣu vicitya dhīrāḥ
pretyāsmāl lokād amṛtā bhavanti

> The sage who leaves this relative and dual world, seeing the Self in every creature, attains immortality.
>
> (*Kena Upanishad*, 2.5b)

"What can cause suffering or illusion to the enlightened ones...?"

I have been asked many times if so-and-so is enlightened. I have even been asked if I am myself enlightened. My answer is that neither I nor anyone else has ever been enlightened, because enlightenment is the disappearance of the ego as a phenomenon. To think that someone can become enlightened is like believing that after turning on a light, darkness will still be there as a kind of enlightened darkness. As we all know, when a light is turned on, darkness disappears, since its very nature is the absence of light. Likewise, the egoic phenomenon is ignorance of what we really are; enlightenment is nothing but the complete extinction of this ignorance. Upanishadic seekers finally recognize themselves, their authentic nature, and what they really are as the very essence of splendor and the golden veil, just like every experience. According to the Vedantic message, you are both the problem and the solution; therefore, the search for Truth begins and ends in you.

There are many states prior to enlightenment, *savikalpa-samādhi*, which comprises *savitarka-samādhi*, *savicāra-samādhi*, *sānanda-samādhi*, and *sāsmitā-samādhi*. Then, we have *nirvikalpa-samādhi*, *sahaja-samādhi*, and, finally, *dharma-megha-samādhi*. The difference between the first and the last state is intimately related to the degree of the dissolution of the ego or subject. At least up to the level *sāsmitā-samādhi*, although objective duality has been largely overcome, there is still a fairly significant presence of the ego or subject. Only with the renunciation of both the object and the subject can relative duality be completely overcome. By transcending both facets of duality, true awakening to the Absolute occurs. This means dying as a subject in space-time to be reborn as eternal subjectivity. It means losing ourselves in order to find ourselves.

There is a great difference between Truth seekers and enlightenment hunters. Truth seekers ask what Truth or reality is; hunters ask how they can obtain, achieve, and maintain this experience. True *sādhakas* ask themselves what or who they are; enlightenment hunters ask how they can obtain God. Seekers want to be; hunters want to acquire. From the egoic perspective, our value in the marketplace of society increases when we possess more. To access the Absolute, one needs to transcend the subject–object duality. No matter how pleasurable it is to possess something, it will unfailingly come with its opposite. No matter how valuable it is, as long as we remain within the limits of duality, its counterpart will always be present.

The cause of suffering lies in our self-perception. We

see ourselves as isolated entities whose goals conflict with those of the Whole. Most of our desires and ambitions are in conflict with the flow of life. Just as a drop of water will suffer as long as it desires go against the current of the river, humans will continue to suffer as long as they resist the powerful flow of life. Since it is a contraction, the ego is seriously threatened by relaxation. As the relaxation of the wave implies its disappearance in the ocean, relaxing the "I" means it dissolves into consciousness. Total surrender implies acceptance, relaxation, and flowing with the Whole.

The root of our suffering is ignorance of what we really are. Kept in the dark by this ignorance, we only perceive limitations. Any restriction means pain and suffering. Supposed happiness, so sought after in our society, is nothing more than an effort to escape this feeling of limitation.

"...who only perceive unity wherever they look."

Before creation, nothing existed but God. Clearly, lacking raw material, God could only create from himself. The universe, with all its contents, is nothing but divinity. Reality is constituted by a great diversity of aspects of the same divine reality. To grasp this, it is essential to bear in mind three fundamental principles: 1) every effect has a cause, 2) all effects are the same cause that manifest as different forms, and 3) if the cause of the effect is eliminated, the effect is also eliminated.

To explain with an analogy, we could say that water is the cause and the sea, with it waves, bubbles, and foam, is the effect. According to the first principle, all manifestations in the sea share the same cause: water. If we look around us, we perceive the diversity but there is a single cause. The second principle says that all forms are manifestations of the same water. This leads us to the conclusion that we are the expression of the primordial cause, or *sarva-kāraṇa-kāraṇam*, manifesting in a myriad of forms. The third principle indicates that, if water were extracted, there would be no sea. That is, without the Self there would be no cosmic manifestation.

The primordial cause of the universe is consciousness or God. Only the Self really is. The phenomenal world is nothing but Brahman manifesting itself in a multiplicity of names and forms. But in the experience of the Self, all objects lose their distinctions and dissolve into the substratum of the world, which is the one reality.

Such a primordial cause of life is sought by both religion and science. Science's search is objective, while religion explores the subjective. Only through subjectivity is it possible to access reality. Awakening to consciousness is possible only through spirituality.

Within a dualistic perception, subject and object are interdependent, because the nature of the object depends on the observation carried out by the subject. When you look at John, he is the object as long as you consider yourself to be the subject. But when John looks at you, he sees you as the object and he thinks he is the subject. The object would not be an object if it were not observed by a subject. If the mental inclination to differentiate between the subject and the diversity of objects is restrained, conceptualizations can be prevented from emerging. By restricting the manifestation of conceptualizations and definitions, the fixed limits between subject and object disappear and both are integrated into the Absolute, non-dual reality.

Thought places illusory limits on consciousness, creating the idea of a subject, or "I," as the basis of an individual personality. This separate "I" is a localization of consciousness and the foundation of the dual dimension. Based on this idea, the mind constructs a world of opposites such as attachment and hatred, happiness and suffering. Consciousness is the infinite space where experience takes place. In the dual and relative dimension, consciousness has the opportunity to perceive itself. In the absolute non-dual dimension, the Self is intangible as an object, but can be realized as the original subjectivity. If in the relative reality the Self is perceived, in the non-dual one is the Self.

The first step is renouncing objects and transcending them, but later, true renunciation is about the subject. Renouncing the object without transcending the subject is like extracting an infected tooth and leaving the root in place. Without going beyond what we think we are, renouncing what we think we possess will be incomplete.

Egoic duality, like a coin, has two sides. It is impossible to renounce one side and keep the other. Even if we hide one side, it will continue to be present. Most people try to achieve and maintain only one side of the coin. Although we strive only for happiness, sadness will come too. If we achieve pleasure, pain will also come. Every gain is accompanied by loss. What is more difficult than giving up what we have gained is transcending the one who gains or the subject. True renunciation means tossing the coin out and getting rid of it altogether.

Enlightenment means fully recognizing that both subject and object are illusionary aspects of the same non-dual reality. Enlightenment is the realization that our true nature is consciousness, which is the raw material of both subject and object.

Mantra 8

स पर्यगाच्छुक्रमकायमव्रणमस्नाविरꣳ शुद्धमपापविद्धम् ।
कविर्मनीषी परिभूः स्वयम्भूर्याथातथ्यतोऽर्थान्व्यदधाच्छाश्वतीभ्यः
समाभ्यः ॥ ८॥

sa paryagāc chukram akāyam avraṇam asnāviram śuddham apāpa-viddham kavir manīṣī paribhūḥ svayambhūr yāthātathyato 'rthān vyadadhāc chāśvatībhyaḥ samābhyaḥ

The Ātman pervades everything. It is radiant, incorporeal, devoid of muscles, pure, immaculate, self-created, and all-embracing. It is the omniscient seer and it is self- sufficient. It has established laws and duties since time immemorial.

COMMENTARY:

In this mantra, the sage's efforts to describe the indescribable continue. Now we will look into some of the terms that the *ṛṣi* uses in this verse:

Paryagāt

Paryagāt means "all-pervading." The term refers to the limitless nature of the Ātman. Permeating everything, it resides in all things and all beings, even in us as the essence of who we are. *Paryagāt* cannot be accessed with thought. The limited nature of the mind prevents it from comprehending the limitless. Therefore, it is impossible to define or conceptualize ultimate reality.

The ancient Mosaic tradition is characterized by a radical rejection of idolatry. As an example, we read in Leviticus (26:1): "You shall not make idols for yourselves, or set up for yourselves carved images or pillars, or place figured stones in your land to worship upon, for I am the Lord your God." We find similar claims in the scriptures of the religions derived from the Hebrew revelation, that is, Christianity and Islam. In its simplest and most basic meaning, an idol is a representation, image, or symbol of divinity that it is worshipped through. It is a limited symbol of the limitless, a finite image of infinity. The Mosaic tradition disapproves of referring to such symbols as if they were what they symbolize, that is, treating a limited representation as if it were unlimited.

Idols begin as ideas, images, or mental objects that are then verbalized and then finally, are sculpted. But the Torah does not refer only to physical idols made of clay, wood, metal, or stone, but to psychological idolatry. This a mental and linguistic idolatry that manufactures idol-ideas or idol-concepts. In reality, every word and idea by which we refer to Ātman—soul, Self, Truth, consciousness, enlightenment, or God—is not real but is only an objective and limited verbal representation of the infinite subjectivity.

Enlightened beings who attempt to define Truth are aware of the absurdity of the endeavor. It is simply irrational to undertake the task of describing the indescribable or conceptualizing limitless subjectivity. It is understandable that, throughout history, many awakened beings have chosen to remain silent, omitting explanations, ideas, or concepts about the Absolute. Some authentic disciples have followed the silence of their masters and adopted it as if it were the definition of Truth. The Upanishadic sages, on the other hand, tried to verbalize the mystery. Their descriptions, though imperfect, may be of some benefit.

From another perspective, we can say that while enlightened masters have emanated from Truth, institutionalized religion has been born from definitions of Truth. For centuries, the phenomenon of organized religion has offered only notions, concepts, ideas, opinions, conjectures, and beliefs that help sell false conceptualizations of Truth. If they were true descriptions as they claim, they would all be the same. But these distortions vary greatly because they are influenced by different cultures and traditions. In contrast, the Upanishadic sages do not offer definitions, but descriptions of transcendental experience. They may be of some use to sincere seekers because they offer intuitive glimpses of the Self.

The term *paryagāt* means "unlimited or omnipresent." To define Ātman, I turn to Pascal's famous phrase used by Borges and so many others: "It is a circle whose circumference is not located anywhere, while its center or axis is everywhere." Being limitless, it is impossible to place Ātman in a specific location, which is why the Torah refers to God as *Ha Makom*, or "the Place." God is not in one place, but it is the place par excellence, where all things and all beings are.

Śukram

Śukram means "radiant." The Self is light, that is, the light of intelligence, observation, and consciousness. In the Bible, we read, "Your life will be brighter than the noonday. Even darkness will be as bright as morning" (Job, 11:17). In the New Testament, Jesus proclaims: "I am the light of the world. Whoever follows me will never walk in darkness, but will have the light of life" (John, 8:12). In the Qur'an, in Surah *An-Nur*, or 'of the Light,' we read: "Allāh is the Light of the heavens and the earth. His Light (in the Universe) may be likened to a niche wherein is a lamp, and the lamp is in the crystal which shines in star-like brilliance. It is lit from (the oil) of a blessed olive tree that is neither eastern nor western. Its oil well night glows forth (of itself) though no fire touched it: Light upon Light. Allāh guides to His Light whom He wills. Allāh sets forth parables to make people understand. Allāh knows everything" (*Surah An-Nur*, 24:35).

The nature of light has been an enigma that has occupied the scientific community for generations. Science understands light as a form of electromagnetic radiation visible to our eyes, and as such, it is the closest thing to pure energy. Light is one form of displaced energy. Light waves are a form of electromagnetic radiation, since they come from vibrating electric and magnetic fields.

In general, matter is identified by its objective physical properties. The most common definition of matter is "anything that has mass and occupies a place in space." For example, we would say that a book is matter because it has mass and occupies space. However, when we review this definition according to quantum mechanics, concepts such as "possessing mass" or "occupying space" are different from our empirical experience.

Another definition of matter would be: "matter is made up of what atoms and molecules are made of." However, there are substances made of the same basic components that are not formed into atoms or molecules. For example, white dwarf matter is typically made of carbon and oxygen nuclei in a sea of degenerate electrons.

At an even deeper level, atoms are made up of protons and neutrons, which in turn are made up of quarks and the force fields that bind them together, or gluons. Early definitions of matter were based on its basic constituents. If we place it on the scale of elementary particles, our earlier definition will read as follows: "ordinary matter is everything that is made up of elementary particles, or fermions, namely quarks and leptons." The search for the basic components of matter has led us to more and more elementary entities, from the molecule to the atom, to the nucleus and electrons, to nucleons, and finally to quarks, in a long process that science is still far from completing. According to several scientists, the foundation of our universe is not only matter or energy, but light, which can behave as a particle or wave, as matter or energy. There are those who have argued—such as Aristotle, Newton, Descartes, or Einstein—that light is made up of particles. However, for other researchers—such as Fresnel, Young, Maxwell, and Huygens—light is a wave. This dual behavior is a quantum phenomenon called wave–corpuscle or wave–particle duality, which has been empirically corroborated. According to this phenomenon, particles may exhibit typical wave-like behavior in some experiments, while appearing as compact, localized particles in others. Sometimes light behaves as matter and sometimes as energy. Thus, according to wave–particle duality, there are no fundamental differences between waves and particles, since one can behave like the other and vice versa.

A group of physicists claimed to have discovered the method for transforming light into matter. These experiments empirically demonstrated the famous theory called the "Breit–Wheeler process," formulated in 1934 by scientists Gregory Breit and John A. Wheeler. They suggested transforming light into matter through the simultaneous destruction of two photons, which would create an electron and a positron. This theory is now a reality, thanks to the demonstration carried out at the Imperial College London, and the results were published in *Nature Photonics*. One of the co-authors is Professor Steve Rose, who states that after eighty years, they have managed to confirm the reality of this theory. In the words of Professor Rose: "This is a pure demonstration of Einstein's famous equation relating energy and mass: $E=mc^2$, which tells us how much energy is produced when matter is converted into energy. We are doing the same, but in reverse: converting photon energy into mass, meaning, $m=E/c^2$."

The experiment went through two phases. The first used a high intensity laser, capable of accelerating electrons to close to the speed of light, that shot the electrons a sheet of gold. This created a beam of photons a billion times more energetic than visible light. In the second phase, a high-energy laser was fired into a vacuum onto the inner surface of the gold, creating a thermal radiation field and thus generating light similar to that emitted by stars. Next, the photon beam from the first phase was directed through the center of the container used in the second phase, in order to collide the photons from both sources. This formed detectable electrons and positrons. The authors of the study claim to have been surprised to discover that the process provided the conditions for the creation of a photon collider.

However, the reality is that light, physical matter, and its density are only an optical illusion, an idea, a concept. If we observe matter closely, at a certain point we will transcend the physical plane and find only light, which has a reality that is unquestionable, more so than any physical form or object. To the extent that we try to penetrate deeper and deeper levels of "solid matter," instead of density we find light. Consequently, objective material existence is only apparent because, ultimately, physical objects are just condensed light, without which nothing of what we perceive in our empirical reality would exist. Meditation is about transcending ourselves as physical bodies and going beyond the mind and emotions in pursuit of our authentic subjectivity. It is allowing the revelation of the light of consciousness in the depths of our inner self.

It is impossible to perceive the light of the Self within the superficial empirical world of names and forms. In the relative and dual dimension, instead of illuminating, we hide the darkness. What we call light in this world is merely an effort to cover the darkness. On the relative plane, we do not turn on the light, but only conceal the darkness. What is perceived in the objective world is not light; true light resides in the innermost recesses of our being. The surface is dark; the depths are radiant.

When light hits an opaque object, it bounces off the object and changes direction. This phenomenon is called *reflection*. Objects reflect part of the light that hits them. These light waves, at different frequencies, reach our retinas and allow us to see objects in color. The fact is that no one has ever perceived light directly. By stating that the room is illuminated, I am really only stating that I can see and I am not blind. It is impossible to see light directly; we only perceive illuminated objects. Thus, light is only an inference or deduction and not a direct experience. It is only possible to see light directly in the depths of our inner self. Such clarity is one of the multiple manifestations of the inner light that illuminates our dreams. That is why those who act from the deepest levels of consciousness manifest greater clarity. That clarity expressed in every word, argument, or look attracts, fascinates, captivates, and enchants us; it awakens a certain nostalgia because it is the very essence of what we are.

We are localized light and luminous waves of clarity. In the superficial dimension of shadows, all light is temporary and relative, while darkness is eternal. On the superficial plane, light can be eliminated by destroying its source and darkness can only be covered momentarily. If every source of light in the universe were eliminated, a vast ocean of darkness would remain. Where night rules, we can try to hide darkness by turning on the light, but we can never eradicate it. However, in our inner world, it is just the opposite: light is eternal and darkness is temporary. No matter how dark our activities are, they do not dim the inner light of consciousness. Even if we make mistakes and behave poorly, our actions do not affect the purity and clarity of consciousness.

Neither darkness on the surface nor light within have cause or origin. This world consists of the dimension of darkness, while light belongs to the interior. Neither the outer darkness nor the inner light comes from a specific source. Consequently, it is impossible to eliminate them. Both originate from the omnipresent Ātman who resides simultaneously everywhere and nowhere. This world is made up of the dimension of darkness or absence of light. The spiritual path leads us toward the dimension of light without origin.

न तद्भासयते सूर्यो न शशाङ्को न पावकः ।
यद्गत्वा न निवर्तन्ते तद्धाम परमं मम ॥

na tad bhāsayate sūryo
na śaśāṅko na pāvakaḥ
yad gatvā na nivartante
tad dhāma paramaṁ mama

Neither the sun nor the moon nor fire can illuminate that supreme abode of mine. Having gone there, one does not return to this material world again.

(Bhagavad Gita, 15.6)

Akāyam

Akāyam means "incorporeal." Expressions such as incorporeal, devoid of muscles, pure, and immaculate point to the purity of consciousness, which lacks qualities and is free from the limits imposed by a certain form. Many human beings believe they are a body. They consider themselves Chilean, Russian, or Ecuadorian, according to the geographical place where their body manifested. Due to such bodily identification, they seek happiness by only trying to satisfy their physical demands. In such a situation, life does not deserve to be called *human*.

आहारनिद्राभयमैथुनानि समान्यमेतत्पशुभिर्नराणाम् ।
ज्ञानंनराणामधिको विशेषो ज्ञानेन हीना पशुभिः समानाः ॥

āhāra-nidrā-bhaya-maithunāni
sāmānyam etat paśubhir narāṇām
jñānaṁ narāṇām adhiko viśeṣo
jñānena hīnāḥ paśubhiḥ samānāḥ

The activities of eating, sleeping, mating, and defending are shared by animals and human beings. Human beings are considered superior only when they inquire about the absolute Truth, otherwise they are just like animals.

(*Hitopadeśa*, 0.25)

Trying to attain bliss, we provide comforts to the body. Logically, these efforts will end in frustration because we will only achieve pleasure. Bodily identification has been instilled in us from our earliest childhood. This mental and emotional interpretation rules our lives. To transcend it, we must adopt a new perspective on our physical dimension. Instead of identifying with our form, we can place ourselves in the position of its observer. By being the witness, we will not live from the conviction that we are the body, but we will be aware of the body. Just as identification has made us believe we are a body, observation allows us to adopt the perspective of being aware of it. By clearly differentiating between the two experiences—between being the body and observing it—we remain observers of the body.

What observes the body is knowledge or perception. Our next step will be to expand observation to include thoughts or mind, sensations or body, and perception or the universe. As we become conscious, we will see that mental and physical activity, as well as perception itself, are situated in us. We are of the same substance and raw material. The sea is water, and therefore, all the forms that the sea acquires, such as waves, bubbles, or foam, are also water. Likewise, everything that appears in consciousness is consciousness.

We are the body, yet not only the body. We are the totality of our experience. In fact, we are the body, the mind, perceptions, and everything that is smelled, touched, tasted, seen, and heard. As consciousness, we share the same substance as sensations, thoughts, and perceptions. We, as pure consciousness, are made of the same substance as our experience. We are not just this bag of flesh and bones that we have accepted as our body, but the totality of universal experience. To experience that we are the body is part of reality; however, to believe that we are only the body is an illusion.

The path to Truth is to stop identifying with the mind and body. To be the Self, or our authentic nature, means transcending such limiting identifications. It is possible to transcend them through observation. It may seem artificial at first, but in time we will discover that it is completely natural. Observation will become the background of our life and we will recover our original identity. We will even retain the perspective of observation during our dreams. Our identification with the body will not cease, but it will expand until we identify with the Whole.

Svayambhūr

Svayambhūr means "self-created." The law of cause and effect is based on the idea that every action provokes a reaction, and vice versa. That is to say, every effect is caused by a prior action. When cause A happens, effect B, or a variety of effects B1, B2 and B3, take place. Likewise, a phenomenon can have several causes: B occurred because A1, A2, and A3 occurred before.

The law of cause and effect pertains to the relative reality, where time and space exist. From a dual perspective, everything we observe in objective reality has a cause. The only thing that lacks a beginning, and therefore a cause, is consciousness itself. Whenever we want to explore an object, we are interested in its origin. To get to know people better, it helps to visit their family or learn about their parents. Although all things and all beings have a cause, we understand that there must be a first cause, which is not preceded by any previous cause. This first cause, the cause of all causes, cannot come from anything or anyone. Consciousness alone has no cause and consequently, it is not an effect. It was never born and will never die, since it is indestructible. Everything that has a beginning also has an end; everything that begins ends. Since it is indestructible, we can assume that consciousness has no beginning.

अक्षरं ब्रह्म परमं स्वभावोऽध्यात्ममुच्यते ।
भूतभावोद्भवकरो विसर्गः कर्मसंज्ञितः ॥

akṣaraṁ brahma paramaṁ
svabhāvo 'dhyātmam uchyate
bhūta-bhāvodbhava-karo
visargaḥ karma-saṁjñitaḥ

Śrī Bhagavān said, "The Supreme, the indestructible is Brahman; its manifestation is *adhyātma*, the Self; the creative process by which all beings are created is called *karma*."

(Bhagavad Gita, 8.3)

The law of cause and effect only exists in the dual and relative dimension. Our inner world is free of causes and effects. Awakening means opening our eyes to non-causal reality.

Although consciousness is not an effect, a wide variety of causes can be purchased in the spiritual marketplace. There are countless techniques for attaining enlightenment. But if there were a method with the result of attaining God, the method would be a cause and God its effect. However, to know God means to know that which is causeless. As long as we look for causes and reasons, we are moving in the relative and dual world. When we find an authentic master, we begin to move in a dimension devoid of cause.

We try to find causes for everything that happens to us in life and, if we do not find them, we imagine them. We feel insecure if we fail to find the reasons for the events that happen to us. Believing ourselves responsible for the situations that we face, we look for the reasons for our supposed behavior. But it is impossible for us to identify the cause of love. I will say in the purest style of Lao-Tzu's *Tao Te Ching*: if you can identify the cause of love, you can be sure that it is not love. Love is invisible and it only lets us perceive the consequences. Likewise, it is impossible to directly see spiritual awakening, we can only see the symptoms. The cause of enlightenment is unattainable. Some say God is love, and perhaps it is because neither have cause nor effect.

The encounter between master and disciple is totally

different from what we consider a relationship in the West. Relationships belong to the dual dimension. Cause and effect are part of a superficial relationship. Communion, on the other hand, is related to the spirit. Observing the master, we realize that something has happened to him or her, but we cannot say exactly what. The awareness and connection of what is happening in the master will produce a response within us. That response is not an effect because the awakening of the master is not the cause of the disciple awakening. In the dimension of the soul, instead of cause and effect, there is simultaneous communion. Simultaneity can only take place with communion, and it manifests when you are synchronized with a phenomenon that inspires you, such as a sunset, the stars, a bird, or a smile. You become accessible and vulnerable to that phenomenon and a response arises from deep within you.

In Hebrew, the language of the Bible, the word for response is *teshuvah*. This is interesting because it is composed of the word *lashuv* ("to go back or to return") and the final letter *he*, which symbolizes divinity. Therefore, to respond would be something like "to return to God." This carries a profound message. Although the Torah does offer intellectual answers, these are not the answers that Truth seekers long for. Authentic and sincere seekers go in search of answers that emerge from within as they synchronize with the mystery of the Torah. This answer is a return to the place we have never left. An answer is triggered from within, responding simultaneously and in absolute harmony with the phenomenon in question. However, such a response has not been caused by your vulnerability nor by the sunset, nor by the bird nor by the smile. The response is born from the depths of your soul so it is not an effect. This sacred book speaks of the real and true, of the eternal and infinite, and something awakens within you.

Masters play their melody and make your soul sing, but their melody is not the cause, nor is your soul's song the effect. The encounter between master and disciple is simultaneous synchronization. If singing were only an effect, everyone would sing at the sound of that melody. Enlightened gurus are equally available to all their disciples. However, disciples evolve at their own pace and proportionally to their openness and accessibility to the master.

Masters are exalted if their disciples become enlightened. This glorification is undeserved because the master is not the cause nor is the disciple's enlightenment the effect. All the merit belongs to the disciples and not the gurus. It is the disciples who have opened themselves, lowered their defenses, and made themselves accessible and vulnerable, making it possible for the response to manifest.

"It has established laws and duties since time immemorial."

This last sentence suggests that consciousness expresses

itself as cosmic order. Consciousness is the essence of all that is. Therefore, there is no real difference between consciousness and the objective universe. Mind, body, and world are, in fact, different shades of one and the same consciousness. Lastly, we only need to understand how it is possible that the laws and order governing the cosmos can be real if they are related to interaction or objective diversity. Within a dream, the laws of nature resemble those of the waking state. But in a dream, it is possible to fly without wings or cross the ocean in a paper boat. Upon awakening, we realize that all these laws were real within the dream but are unreal while awake. They are only part of the dream reality and were always the experience of the dreamer. However, we only become aware of this upon awakening. Similarly, from a transcendental perspective, the laws of the waking state will be perceived as those of the dream only after awakening. What the Upanishad states in this sentence is that the source and origin, the substance or raw material, as well as the destiny of everything apparent, is only the Self or consciousness.

Mantra 9

अन्धं तमः प्रविशन्ति येऽविद्यामुपासते ।
ततो भूय इव ते तमो य उ विद्यायाꣳ रताः ॥

andhaṁ tamaḥ praviśanti
ye 'vidyām upāsate
tato bhūya iva te tamo
ya u vidyāyāṁ ratāḥ

Those who are dedicated to the cultivation of ignorance (*avidyā*) will fall into the region of blinding darkness, but those who are attached to knowledge (*vidyā*) will fall into even greater darkness.

COMMENTARY:

Although the word *avidyā* is usually translated as "ignorance," its literal meaning is "no wisdom"; that is, *avidyā* does not indicate something that exists, but something that is absent. In the Tibetan language, the term *ignorance* (*ma rig pa*) is also composed of the negative prefix (*ma* instead of *a* in Sanskrit) preceding the term *truth* (*rig pa*). For Vedanta, *avidyā* is not an antonym of wisdom, because it is not the opposite of it. Just as darkness is the absence of light and cold the absence of heat, *avidyā* is the absence of wisdom. The nature of *avidyā* is apparent and, therefore, lacks an autonomous existence. There is no point in dealing with what is illusory, because only what exists is operational. Consequently, we can only refer to the presence or absence of knowledge.

Ignorance is *māyā*, "that which is not" or "that which does not exist." *Māyā* is *avidyā* on the universal plane, while *avidyā* is the same illusion on the individual plane. If ignorance were real, then acquiring knowledge would cover it with information. Ignorance would remain beneath knowledge. Instead of eliminating ignorance, knowledge would only cover it, so that ignorance would still be the basis of acquired knowledge. However, knowledge eradicates ignorance, just as light dispels darkness. Like a powerful acid, when what is real appears, it dissolves what is unreal. In the words of Confucius, "Ignorance is the night of the mind, but a night without moon or stars."

In the context of mantras 9, 10, and 11 of this Upanishad, the Vedantic terms *avidyā* and *vidyā* can be confusing so they need to be clarified. Like *veda* and *vijñāna*, *vidyā* comes from the root *vid* meaning "to know." These Sanskrit terms have much broader implications than their English or Spanish equivalents. They have been used in different ways throughout the Vedic literature. *Vidyā* refers to "meditation" in various Upanishads, while in yoga terminology this is *dhyāna*. In the context of this verse, *vidyā* refers to an attitude of internalization or introspection that aims at perceiving the unmanifested or the subjective. *Avidyā* and *vidyā* denote two diametrically opposed dispositions. The former corresponds to an active and extroverted attitude, the latter to a passive and introspective one. *Avidyā* is an externalization while *vidyā* an internalization. The former points to the objective, while the latter aims for the depths of our subjectivity. *Avidyā* refers to a segregationist disposition directed toward multiplicity and *vidyā* denotes the appreciation of what cannot be apprehended through the senses.

Extroverts tend to be assertive and have various social skills. Because they communicate well what they think and feel, they are able to make friends easily. They like changes and respond skillfully to any situation. They are energetic and active. They enjoy new activities and are constantly on the move. However, extroverts pay more attention to their external experiences than their inner world. Their main interests are their surroundings and their social life. They experience the need to socialize, to be surrounded by other people, and to attend social gatherings. They tend to be impulsive, in other words, they make decisions and act without reflecting.

For Vedanta, ignorance does not mean just not knowing, but implies a cognitive externalization that is related to the consciousness of diversity or objective knowledge. *Avidyā* manifests as admiration toward names and forms and an adoration of all that is objective. Ignorance is expressed as surrender and giving in to relative reality. According to this, culture, economics, science, and technology, and in general, all intellectual knowledge, can be considered different expressions of *avidyā*. If we pay attention, we will see that ignorant people are unaware of their own ignorance. They may be informed, but they are ignorant because they are unaware of what they do not know. Since activity belongs to the phenomenal world, *avidyā* is synonymous with movement, action, or karma. Time, space, form, and motion can only exist on the basis of *avidyā*. Consequently, activity and the doer, or *ahaṅkāra*, can only stand on the foundation of *avidyā*.

Venerating relative reality originates from *avidyā*. This fervor is expressed as seeking bliss through the senses, which may include prayers, sacrifices, and rituals performed for temporary worldly benefits. This demand only leads to frustration since, while it is possible to feel happiness through the body, it is impossible to experience bliss. The following verse explains who can attain bliss.

द्वावेव चिन्तया मुक्तौ परमानन्द आप्लुतौ ।
यो विमुग्धो जडो बालो यो गुणेभ्यः परं गतः ॥

dvāveva cintayā muktau
paramānanda āplutau
yo vimugdho jaḍo bālo
yo guṇebhyaḥ paraṁ gataḥ

> In this world, two types of people are free from all anxiety and merged with great bliss: one who is a mentally retarded childish fool and one who has approached the transcendental and is beyond the three modes of material nature.
>
> (*Śrīmad-bhāgavatam*, 11.9.4)

The *Śrīmad-bhāgavatam* states that only enlightened beings and idiots can be blissful in this world. Only those in the middle suffer. This recalls the *beinoni*, or "mediocre" in Hebrew, from the book *Tanya*.

What we call *happiness* is nothing more than a temporary relief from suffering. Our so-called happiness depends on previous afflictions. Without feeling sadness first, we would not experience happiness. As the psychiatrist Carl Jung, "the term *happiness* would lose all meaning if it were not compensated by sadness." We enjoy sleeping because sleep relieves fatigue. We indulge in a meal only after experiencing hunger. The company of friends or a partner brings us joy us because we have been lonely. Certainly, we will not find any pleasure in a glass of water unless we are thirsty. If we look closely, we notice that the pleasure that accompanies each experience is proportional to the suffering it alleviates. The supposed pleasure can become suffering if it lacks its corresponding previous pain. Forcing a satisfied person who has just had lunch to eat more food would be real torture. For someone who has drunk his fill, one more glass of water would be a punishment. Likewise, after a good night's sleep, staying in bed can be a source of anxiety. In conclusion, without the absence of pleasure, it would be impossible to enjoy.

Moreover, the more available the source of pleasure, the less pleasure it will give us. If we are in the company of our best friends all the time, we will long for solitude. If we eat our favorite food for breakfast, lunch, and dinner, we will end up detesting it. Any enjoyment or happiness requires a temporary lapse that allows us to perceive its absence. There is no object or activity that gives pleasure continuously with the same intensity. This cycle is called *bhoga-tyāga* in Sanskrit and consists of pleasure followed by abstinence. This cycle can be seen in our life of work and vacation, waking and sleeping, striving and resting, eating and fasting, and so on. There is no activity, object, or person that we can enjoy with the same intensity on a permanent basis. It is interesting that human beings dream of a constant happiness free of suffering. We desire an eternal and ever intensifying happiness. It is strange that, although we know that bliss does not exist on the relative plane, we seek it persistently.

The reason is that our true nature is absolute bliss, or *ānanda*. What we really are is absolute bliss, which is independent of an opposite in the form of pain or suffering and is beyond pleasure and joy.

"... they will enter a region of blinding darkness..."

Darkness has a profound meaning in the context of Vedantic revelation. To explain it, we will use the well-known analogy of the rope and the snake. In the darkness of night, a person stumbles over a rope and mistakes it for a snake. Such misperception leads to negative feelings such as anxiety, panic, or distress. All of these feelings are very real. But with the light of dawn, such feelings fade away as the error is perceived. The rope represents consciousness or our true reality. Mistaking the rope for a snake is the illusion. The darkness symbolizes our limitation in recognizing consciousness, which does not allow a clear perception of what is, as it is. As long as the darkness persists, we will be unable to see that the rope is just a rope and there never was a snake. In the shadows, we stumble, we collide, we fall, we mistake friends for enemies and vice versa.

"... but those who are attached to knowledge (*vidyā*) will fall into even greater darkness."

Vidyā (*jñānam*) is the knowledge accumulated by the knower (*jñātṛ*) about the empirical environment within the relative context. The verse refers to *vidyā* as an introspective attitude. Choosing introspection and rejecting worldly externalization is a reaction that deepens differences, conflicts, and finally, darkness. Every choice will always be partial. Vedanta aims at totality.

Countries try to establish social or legal order in different ways. The problem is that those who suffer from internal disorder cannot create external order. A society with internal conflicts can never live in harmony. We have to grasp the totality of existence in order to understand the conflict and thus be able to overcome it. Observing life in its entirety is a difficult task for human beings who suffer from internal fractures that lead them to conflict, disorder, and confusion. This inner conflict expresses itself as aggression and violence for individuals and as crime and wars for the collective.

Human beings are trapped in the division between activity and meditation, that is, externalization and internalization. However, both the external and the internal consist only of interpretations. Both directions are merely apparent conceptions without real foundations. Conceptions stem from thought, which is based on fragmentation. The mind projects division and conflict; it is not integral because it only knows how to move between polarities. Because of its partial nature, peace and harmony cannot reign in the mind.

Observation and thought never meet: thought arises only in the absence of observation. In fact, thought is an obstacle to observation. Only by observing without thought intervening, is it possible to clearly see mental structure. The dualities subject–observer and object–observed originate from a lack of attention. We must observe the movement of thought, but without adopting the position of subject–observer, distanced from the object–observed. The observer disappears when the observation is free of knowledge, previous understanding, judgment, or preconceived ideas about what is observed. Observing the mental process without rejecting what is observed eliminates the intrusion of thought. Attentive observation is deeply loving. Only by observing with love, and without projecting our mental content, is it possible to perceive existence in its totality.

Any attempt to divide life between action and meditation, extroversion and introversion, or material and spiritual, leads to conflict, disorder, and darkness. There are those who focus their attention on external reality and believe that only empirical reality exists. On the other hand, there are those who opt for a life of introspection in which only the inner world matters. For the former, the body is the most important thing, while for the others, it is the soul. However, human beings are both body and soul. The body is the material aspect of the soul and the soul is the spiritual aspect of the body. The separation between inner and outer, material or spiritual, comes from the ego. Countless representatives of *avidyā* believe that only matter is real and that consciousness is a byproduct of matter. On the other hand, representatives of *vidyā* and organized religion have thought just the opposite: only the soul and the afterlife are valuable, so they despise the body and the world. However, human beings are organic realities that do not accept divisions. They cannot be understood partially as material or spiritual, but in their totality. Like wheels, humans have a rim and an axle. The body is the rim; the soul is the axle. The rim is superficial and it is impossible to separate it from the axle without destroying the wheel. Both parts form a complete whole that is impossible to break apart.

Human beings are organic realities. Although they are indivisible, they express themselves in different physical, mental, and spiritual ways. Physiological needs are the most immediate and include food, drink, rest, and shelter. Without satisfying our physiological needs, we will not pay attention to higher needs. For example, we will not worry about getting tickets to a concert without having basic food for ourselves and our family. If we suffer from physiological needs, we will lose interest in higher topics such as affection, art, belonging, and recognition. Only after our physical needs have been satisfied will we awaken to our psychological needs. And only after that will we have sincere urges to pray or meditate. Remember that the majority of enlightened beings come from wealthier backgrounds. Jesus was the son of a carpenter, and considering the scarcity of wood in the Middle East, we can guess that this was not an ordinary profession.

Moses grew up in the house of Pharaoh. Kṛṣṇa belonged to the military caste, and Buddha, to royalty. The spiritual path means striving to answer the call of our higher demands, while trying to satisfy the appetite to return to our source and origin. In reality, materialism is the most basic form of spirituality and spiritual life is materialism at its most refined expression. Materialism is the first step on the spiritual path. Spirituality is the very culmination of hedonistic materialism.

Mantra 10

अन्यदेवाहुर्विद्ययाऽन्यदाहुरविद्यया ।
इति शुश्रुम धीराणां ये नस्तद्विचचक्षिरे ॥

anyad evāhur vidyayā
'nyad āhur avidyayā
iti śuśruma dhīrāṇāṁ
ye nas tad vicacakṣire

I have listened from the sages that different results are obtained from the cultivation of knowledge and the cultivation of ignorance.

Commentary:

"I have listened from the sages that" ...

The Sanskrit term *śuśruma* means "I have listened" in the aorist verb form, derived from the root *śru*, which means "to listen." The Upanishadic sages do not teach borrowed theology, but share their own realizations. Instead of repeating the words of their masters by saying "the sages said," they preface these receptive experiences with "I have listened from the sages."

What others think belongs to them and is unrelated to us. Only what we have listened to and assimilated is ours. What we listen to is digested until it becomes part of our own reality. The truths that the Vedantic sages share are not repeated information. They do not preach stale words that someone else said about someone who experienced something. Instead, they generously share silences that they listened to and assimilated at the feet of their masters and discovered as their own. They do not repeat what was said by others many years ago, but they engage us in what they themselves grasped, drank, assimilated, digested, and realized, living in the shadow of the presence of their masters.

Listening and hearing are two different actions. We can hear without the intention of listening, while listening means paying attention. Unlike hearing, the action of listening is voluntary, intentional, and conscious. When we hear, our auditory system detects pressure variations caused by the propagation of sound waves in the air and transforms them into electrical impulses. This information is then transmitted to our brain. We hear noises and listen to what is being said to us. If we listen to our neighbors arguing, we are eavesdropping; otherwise, we only hear them fighting. It is like a speaker who asks someone in the back row if they could hear, to which he replies: "I listened very carefully, but unfortunately I couldn't hear you very well."

The disciple's life is centered on listening to the master. The follower hears; the disciple listens. The difference has to do with quality. What we hear does not affect our daily life and does not change us, but what we assimilate and digest transforms us in a radical way. What we listen to is in accordance with what we are capable of living, while what we hear is only information. When there are sounds but you are not present, you hear; you do not listen. Although many have heard the words of sages, few have listened to them. Those who have heard them will only declaim recycled truths and may even give highly informative lectures and courses. But those who have listened will share the master's presence and soul. The great disciple who wrote this verse does not refer to the teachings of his masters, but to the fact that he was able to listen. To be an academic student, it is enough to hear, but to enter into discipleship it is essential to learn to listen. Anyone who hears is capable of storing enough information and then repeat it in examinations and tests. However, only the listener perceives the spirit that is behind the wisdom. Only a true disciple can listen to the presence of silence.

"...different results are obtained from the cultivation of knowledge and the cultivation of ignorance."

The verse states the implications of cultivating *avidyā* or *vidyā* separately. Each one offers its own advantages and disadvantages. The cultivation of *avidyā* increases our sensory, mental, and intellectual capacities. However, those who follow only the path of active extroversion will find it difficult to recognize consciousness and will not value the soul, spirit, consciousness, or God. Religion and spiritual development will be meaningless to them and every effort to pursue inner evolution will seem like a waste of time. Identifying only with the physical aspect, they will lead a materialistic life centered on the body, mind, senses, and possessions. They will objectify everything, including themselves, and live according to a totally corporeal or materialistic concept of life. They will not only consider themselves a body, but will reduce everything to bodies or objects. Even when cultivators of *avidyā* are in love, they reduce their beloved to an object. The woman reduces her beloved to a husband; the man reduces his beloved to a wife. On the other hand, spiritual people are able to personalize even objects and to enter into communion with their refrigerator, books, and desk.

Cultivating *avidyā* without *vidyā* leads many people

to acquire objects or things without moderation and acquire unnecessary goods. Buying objects causes us pleasure, but if we become attached to them, we fall into addiction. In order to keep up with those around us, we stretch our paychecks to constantly upgrade our computers, cell phones, and cars. The compulsion to buy something before evaluating whether we really need it is a symptom of inner deficiency, caused by cultivating only *avidyā*. Our possessions are a tangible demonstration that we have money. The way to demonstrate power is to possess material objects that express our economic status. In a superficial society, we are measured by what we own and not by who we are. Materialistic societies that are victims of consumerism have the highest levels of depression, addiction, anxiety, obesity, crime, and suicide. Materialism is both the cause and the effect of consumerism. However, this is an illusion, because bliss cannot be purchased.

When faced with the desire to buy, the brain releases a burst of dopamine. The reward is received before the purchase and not with the purchase itself. Because of this pleasurable experience, most people buy the product. The pleasure fades minutes later and we once again have the impulse to buy. The reality is that human beings do not want to possess more for themselves, but only want to have more than others. Lack of internalization makes it difficult to appreciate ourselves. Cultivators of *avidyā* suffer from low self-esteem because it requires an introspective view to discover our inner beauty.

However, by increasing our self-worth through personal development, and not through the acquisition of objects, materialism and consumerism decrease. It is possible to be happy with what we already have, not just by acquiring what we desire.

Technological advances have changed our society. The value we place on basic needs has diminished and the need to consume for no reason has emerged. This increases our dedication to *avidyā* and takes us away from *vidyā*. Work, money, greed, and competition absorb human beings into a routine that is incompatible with introspection. Without valuing inner evolution, economic issues become excessively important. We deceive ourselves into thinking that we will find what we are looking for in the objects we acquire. Without introspection, we cannot reflect on the usefulness of the product we wish to buy and what our real needs are.

Modern society cultivates *avidyā* and, consequently, it is practically impossible to live without consuming. Therefore, I do not condemn the act of consumption itself, but only excessive consumption. We have to buy what is necessary. The problem begins when we acquire things that are unnecessary. There is an immense difference between consumption and consumerism. Consumption sustains the global economy. It is beneficial, as long as it is in harmony with our needs and those of the environment. But our desire to possess objects has promoted an excessive and irresponsible growth of the industrialized world. Excessive materialism affects the environment. The future is in danger unless we develop an ecological consciousness and understand that objects can be recycled to reduce the damage we cause to the planet. People should be educated to consume with balance and responsibility. But without introspection, we even lack awareness of our true needs.

In an excessively extroverted society, mass media plays a fundamental role because it conditions us to work, earn money, and buy things in order to have value in society. Advertising is in the hands of economic interests closely connected to increasing production, which ultimately depends on consumption. The only way to achieve excessive consumption is to create a society where people live to possess. Instead of technology and media serving human beings, they are at the service of profits, which impose an ideology of consumerism.

Humans are transformed into one-dimensional beings and become gears of a great machine that works according to the laws of supply and demand. The gap is widening between the dispossessed and the wealthy in each country, and between poor and rich countries internationally. Despite tremendous technological progress in recent years, the problems afflicting the underdeveloped world have increased. Consumer society places money above human beings, and production above nature; it is fascinated by appearances, status, and possessions. The consumer system wants us to buy first and only then think about the purpose of our purchases. It tries to invade our privacy and enslave us. It does not promote critical thinking nor does it allow spaces for introspection, because this would lead us to reflect.

In a society that cultivates *avidyā*, even spirituality has become institutionalized. It is represented by transnational entities and large structures of power and control. Their original spiritual aspirations have been buried by worldly interests. Organized religion is devoid of spirituality. Like a corpse, it is a body without a soul. In fact, spirituality is not found in temples and rituals, but in the depths of our being.

Consumerism deeply conflicts with the inner quest. It tries to replace "being" with "possessing." This way of life creates a society that leaves no room for the evolution of human values. Our indifference to extreme poverty and our excessive ambition leads us to destroy the planet. In today's global reality, a profound collective reflection is indispensable in order to find solutions. However, in a society that cultivates ignorance, such solutions seem utopian.

Despite the disadvantages, the cultivation of *avidyā* offers certain advantages, such as the development of technology. Human beings have perfected their ability to survive in nature. In fact, all modern instruments are nothing more than extensions of our bodies and abilities. With the rapid advancement of transportation and communications, distances have been reduced, because of fiber optics and satellites. Technological advances have been the unifying element of globalization. By globalization, I mean the reduction of distances between nations, rapid access to information, strong commercial activity between countries, and the ability of superpowers to dominate underdeveloped countries. In a world of constant change, we find such innovations in every corner of our daily lives. However, it is impossible to deny that technology is profoundly changing our perception of the world.

Although we do not all adapt at the same speed, it is interesting to reflect on the extent that technology affects our balance as a society. Computers, cell phones, e-mail, social networks, and artificial intelligence mark our lives because they force us to adapt to technological advances. Technology has changed, but human beings have also changed along with it. We can only hope that technology does not dehumanize us and that it remains at the service of human beings and not the other way around.

Likewise, the cultivation of *vidyā*, or introspection, also has its advantages and disadvantages. The main advantage is that it provides internalization in the form of relaxation, but the exclusive cultivation of introspection limits our development within the world. The main disadvantages come from disregarding what is external in pursuit of what is internal. God is the essence of everything and everyone, therefore, by rejecting matter, we are rejecting God. Those who cultivate *vidyā* interpret spiritual life as a rejection of the world; they see religion as a phenomenon contrary to the world and condemn it. They conceive of religion as a kind of masochism because the attainment of holiness depends on our ability to torture ourselves. For example, they think that religious people must live a life of poverty and that if we possess money, the doors of spiritual life will be closed to us. But for truly religious and spiritual people, there are no boundaries between the material and the spiritual aspects, because they see life as unity.

In conclusion, cultivating *vidyā* and *avidyā* separately yield very different results.

Mantra 11

विद्यां चाविद्यां च यस्तद्वेदोभयꣳ सह ।
अविद्यया मृत्युं तीर्त्वा विद्ययाऽमृतमश्नुते ॥

vidyāṁ cāvidyāṁ ca yas
tad vedobhayaṁ saha
avidyayā mṛtyuṁ tīrtvā
vidyayā'mṛtam aśnute

Only by simultaneously knowing ignorance and knowledge can one overcome the influence of death through ignorance and experiencing immortality through knowledge.

COMMENTARY:

"Can one overcome the influence of death through ignorance."

We have already noted that *avidyā* is related to worldly activity, or karma. Every action is motivated by fear of death. According to Patañjali, this is the essential fear that underlies all fears.

स्वरसवाही विदुषोऽपि तथारूढोऽभिनिवेशः ॥

svarasa-vāhī viduṣo 'pi tathārūḍho 'bhiniveśaḥ

Attachment to life, or fear of death, is established even in the learned ones, since it flows by itself.
(*Yoga Sūtra*, 2.9)

Fear of death torments ignorant and learned people alike. Ignorance about our true nature brings us anguish. On the path of the spirit, we only know what we can put into practice in our lives.

The fear of extinction is the real motivation behind humankind's advancement, in all areas. Human endeavors in various fields of research are aimed at resisting death. Advances in science, technology, medicine, and defense are intended to stop the passage of time, extend life, and protect us from danger. The threat of the end motivates worldly activity in society. Unfortunately, there are very few who act out of inspiration, which is a nobler and higher motivation.

Our society has not been built on a love of life, but a fear of death. This fear motivates us to project ourselves beyond death through our children, to excel in society, and to perpetuate our legacy. This fear drives us to unite in tribes, villages, towns, cities, and nations. We do not create countries motivated by fraternal love, but the fear of perishing. I am sorry to disappoint many of you, but human beings only come together to protect each other. This fear is also the main cause behind religious organizations, each with its own gods, angels, and paradises.

Fearing the end of the body motivates human beings to philosophize, reflect, and speculate on subjects that if they were eternal, they would not care about. Most humans understand immortality as the eternal life of an ego or a personality. With such a precarious understanding of life, it is logical to conclude that the ephemeral nature of life elevates the value of each moment. The writer Jorge Luis Borges expressed this in his short story *The Immortal*. The character in the story is someone who will never die and meets another immortal named Homer, to whom he says:

> Nothing can occur only once; nothing is preciously precarious. The elegiac, the somber, and the ceremonial do not hold for Immortals. Homer and I went our separate ways at the portals of Tangier; I do not think we said goodbye.

Clearly, two immortals do not need to say farewell, because in the course of eternity, they will certainty meet again. Only temporary and transient human beings say, "see you soon, take care, have a great one," because each farewell may be the last one.

In fact, life is only a path that leads to death. Every passing brings sorrow, not only for the deceased but especially for others. When mourning the death of somebody, there is a sense of grief that is stirred by the prospect of our own end. This is wonderfully expressed by John Donne in Meditation XVII of his famous work *Devotions Upon Emergent Occasions*:

> No man is an island, entire of itself; every man is a piece of the continent, a part of the main; if a clod be washed away by the sea, Europe is the less, as well as if a promontory were, as well as if a manor of thy friend's or of thine own were; any man's death diminishes me, because I am involved in mankind, and therefore never send to know for whom the bell tolls; it tolls for thee.

Human society has long perceived death through the wrong prism. Death should not be seen as a final destruction or elimination, but as part of a process of evolutionary renewal. Every moment contains both life and death because renewal is a constant need. We are born with our first inhalation and leave the world with our last exhalation. Life is inhaling; death is exhaling.

With each inhalation we are reborn to life and with each exhalation we die a bit. Every breath contains both inhalation and exhalation because each moment is simultaneous living and dying.

Breathing is a vital process that involves the intake of oxygen into the body and the release of carbon dioxide from the lungs. Both movements are interdependent, because in order to inhale, we must first exhale and vice versa. They do not conflict but rather complement each other in a process of organic renewal. Like inhalation and exhalation, life and death are two aspects of the same process. When observing life through the mind, it is impossible to have a holistic vision of the Whole. The mind perceives polarities in continuous conflict: day and night, positive and negative, feminine and masculine, war and peace, life and death. The Torah teaches that if we look deeply into opposing and even conflicting situations, we will find unity amid apparent contradictions.

בֶּן בַּג בַּג אוֹמֵר: הֲפָךְ בָּהּ וַהֲפָךְ בָּהּ, דְּכֹלָּא בָהּ.
(פרקי אבות ה', כ"ב)

Ben Bag Bag says: "Turn it over, and [again] turn it over, for all is therein."

(*Pirkei Avot*, 5.22)

In the English translation, it is difficult to appreciate the wisdom that this Hebrew phrase conveys. *Hafoch* is translated as "turn over"; however, the word includes the term *hefech*, or "contrary," which hints that if we look at opposites, we will find the Whole. That is to say, the Whole is discovered by observing contradictions. In a moment of mental silence beyond the intellect, in which the Torah is perceived from the soul, whatever seems antagonistic is interdependent, interconnected, and complementary.

The yin–yang symbol is a gift from ancient Chinese philosophy. It contains great wisdom: nature is arranged into pairs of opposing, yet complementary, energies, which coexist in harmony. In the symbol, we see a white fish and a black fish. The white one has a black dot and the black one has a white dot. This shows how these polarities grow, develop, and nurture each other. When we experience deep internalization during meditation, we are white and it is time to hold onto the black dot. We need to allow the black dot to remain and not be consumed by the white fish. We are black when we teach, sing, dance, or paint. In that moment of externalization, we should retain the white dot. The presence of the other polarity keeps us centered. However, if we lose balance, we will fall into darkness.

Big cities are inhabited by many people who do not know how to internalize; monasteries are inhabited by people who do not know how to function in the world. Dance outwardly or meditate inwardly, but always stay in contact with the polarity. Meditate, but do not stop dancing; pray, but do not stop singing; elevate yourself, but do not condemn the world. Realize the One without a second but keep supporting others. Access the Divine without condemning the human. Harmony is the power of the Whole. Therefore, by maintaining the balance, your words and movements will manifest the power of the entire universe.

Many people wonder if there is life after death, but I can assure you that what really matters is that there is life before death. It is in life that we can understand death. We will understand death only after consciously experiencing it. Meditation is like consciously experiencing death while alive, because both death and meditation involve a conscious experience of distancing ourselves from our bodies.

Out of the fear of death, humans have divided life and death; they believe life is positive and death is dramatic. We live escaping death and protecting ourselves from it. However, let me tell you that just as inhalation affects exhalation, our attitude toward death affects our quality of our life. If you are afraid to inhale, you will not be able to exhale and you will suffocate in life. Both inhalation and exhalation, as well as life and death, are interdependent and complementary. If you try to escape death, you will escape life. If you protect yourself from death, you will protect yourself from life. If you try to distance yourself from death, you will distance yourself from life. Whoever fears death, fears life.

Spiritual seekers must cope with the fear of death and the dissolution of their identities. It is understandable to fear the disappearance of whatever defines us as human beings: our names, forms, thoughts, ideas, concepts, conclusions, and emotions. This fear is as a result of entrusting our identity to a set of concepts and sensations. We consider these ideas to be our mind, just as we consider our sensations to be our body. Our original nature has become intermingled with emotions, feelings, and concepts. Our authenticity has become entangled with these phenomena to the extent that it has become entirely eclipsed by them.

As a result of this mistaken identification, we perceive ourselves as a bodily, temporal, and limited entity confined by time and space. Consequently, we live in frustration and constant dissatisfaction. These uncomfortable feelings are a warning that "something is not as it should be." What is happening is that the unlimited and infinite has been confused with the limited and finite. Unlimited consciousness has fallen into a conditioned state. But from the absolute perspective of consciousness, there is no limitation whatsoever. It is the apparent and separate "I" that believes itself to be limited.

To transcend body and mind, we should disconnect our attention from the objective reality we think we know and focus it on the knowledge itself through which we know. By allowing attention to turn toward itself, we will realize that there never was a limited "I" and that we have never ceased to be pure consciousness. Then, fear will disappear because we will see that the loss of our identity is not destruction, but recognition. Instead of disappearing, we recognize that we are eternally conscious beings. This is the true awakening to the reality of our innermost immortality.

These three mantras (9–11) teach us that those who focus their attention on worldly activities and ignore the very essence of life fall into darkness. However, those who only develop internalization and despise action as mundane fall into even greater darkness. For the true sage, action and meditation are not two antagonistic phenomena. Quite the contrary, sages meditate and act at the same time and consider them to be complementary. In fact, both *avidyā* and *vidyā*, action and passivity, externalization and internalization, are two sides of the same coin.

"overcome the influence of death through ignorance…"

Humans need food, water, medicine, and shelter. In the absence of *avidyā*, it would be impossible to survive. Living is more than not dying. All progress in science, medicine, and technology is aimed at saving human beings from death. While science makes it possible to postpone death, it is impossible to experience immortality. Immortality is the aspect of our existence that dwells deep within us, before, during, and after life.

"and experience immortality through knowledge."

Note the subtle difference indicated by the Upanishad: through *avidyā* it is possible to overcome the influence of death, but only through *vidyā* can immortality be attained. The body is only an accumulation of sensations, so perpetuating the body would be like living in an eternal fantasy. Realizing immortality means discovering our eternal aspect, which transcends physical birth and death. What is immortal within us is consciousness. Experiencing immortality means realizing what we really are. Through *vidyā*, it is possible to experience eternity and recognize that we are not just a body, a mind, emotions, nor the idea of "I." We are not just someone but everyone. We are not just something but the Whole or immortality itself.

Most religions teach that the soul is immortal and, therefore, death is not to be feared. However, for many of the faithful, believing in the soul's immortality is nothing more than a consolation for their fear of death. Their minds seek to somehow maintain their attachment to life and they cling to any comforting belief. Religions sell painkillers, telling people not to worry about death because the soul is eternal. Believe me when I say that institutionalized religiosity has not built churches, synagogues, mosques, and temples out of love for God, but out of fear of death. Instead of expressing love and joy, their prayers are contaminated by the dread of death.

Experiencing immortality is very different. It is not about believing in an immortal soul, but realizing that death does not exist because there is no "someone" who can die. There are only sensations, thoughts, and perceptions as shades of one and the same consciousness.

Just as there is no one in life, there will be no one in death. The reality is that only our non-existence as "someone" or "something" can die.

"Only by simultaneously knowing ignorance and knowledge can one overcome the influence of death through ignorance and experience immortality through knowledge."

Both *vidyā* and *avidyā* are very important in the lives of authentic spiritual seekers. The two are intimately connected. We should act with a selfless attitude, giving ourselves to the service of others. Our work should focus not on the product of our efforts, but on offering the results of our activity to the Supreme. Only this fraternal and supportive activity will prepare us for meditation. Through activity motivated solely by love and compassion, the influence of death will be overcome, since all unselfish labor works against the egoic phenomenon and, consequently, eliminates the effects of the idea of death.

In fact, death does not exist, since there is no one who can die. We are not "something" or "someone" and, therefore, there is no death. Death is a mere shadow of the ego. In the same way, the ego is a shadow of what we really are. To escape from the ego is to flee from our own shadow. Trying to destroy the ego is a determined effort to eliminate our shadow. To understand the illusory nature of death, we must understand the egoic phenomenon.

The inexistence of death is revealed by discovering that the ego does not exist. What we really are is existence and eternity. The way to realize this is through observation, which means withdrawing attention from the objects we think we know and directing it toward the knowledge through which we know.

Mantra 12

अन्धं तमः प्रविशन्ति येऽसम्भूतिमुपासते ।
ततो भूय इव ते तमो य उ सम्भूत्याᳬ रताः ॥

andhaṁ tamaḥ praviśanti
ye 'sambhūtim upāsate
tato bhūya iva te tamo
ya u sambhūtyām ratāḥ

Those who worship the manifested enter the region of darkness; even worse happens to the worshippers of the unmanifested.

COMMENTARY:

This mantra begins a triad, mantras 12–14. These mantras restate the same ideas on *vidyā* and *avidyā* that are expressed in mantras 9–11. They emphasize the terms *sambhūti*, or "the manifested" and *asambhūti*, or "the unmanifested," to clarify that they are not opposed but complementary.

Human beings do not perceive reality as it is. They are not observers, but constant interpreters and commentators. Because of our interpretations, we divide existence into *sambhūti* and *asambhūti*. The unmanifested is the aspect of consciousness that has not yet come into existence. The manifested is expressed when consciousness is located in the objective dimension.

Our empirical experience of names and forms is *sambhūti*, or the "manifested": the objective reality on physical, mental, emotional, and energetic levels. The totality of what we think we are is part of *sambhūti*. Even we ourselves as "someone" are part of this objective reality.

Sambhūti is the reality of dissociated entities and objects that appear to be solid. *Sāṅkhya* philosophy posits that the manifested reality is composed of *prakṛti* (primordial matter) and the three *guṇas* (elemental qualities): *sattva, rajas*, and *tamas*. Most human beings only interact with the objective reality around them. Their lives unfold only on the manifested plane.

That which is not expressed in the objective world is called *asambhūtim*, or the "unmanifested." This is the unmanifested aspect that is unknown to us. *Asaṁbhūti* refers to the unmanifested *prakṛti,* the state prior to the manifestation of the world of names and forms. In that state, the *guṇas* are in complete balance. The imbalance between them is what precipitates manifestation.

The text reflects the ancestral debate between loving and knowing, between *bhakti* and *jñāna*. For generations, it has been debated whether it is superior to worship a God with a form or to meditate on the Absolute. The age-old conflict between dualistic personalism and *Advaita* impersonalism debates whether God is *someone* or whether God simply *is*. Thanks to this rivalry, great masters have clarified and enriched our path with schools such Advaita by Ādi Śaṅkarācārya, *Viśiṣṭādvaita* by Rāmānujācārya, *Dvaita* by Madhvācārya, and *Acintya-bhedābheda-tattva* by Caitanya.

"Those who worship the manifested..."

Worship of the manifested means devotion to the personal God, Īśvara, which has a different name in every religion. Īśvara refers to the immanent aspect of God and images of deities that are worshipped in the temple.

Saṁbhūti means *sākāra* (with form) and *asaṁbhūti* is *nirākāra* (formless). These terms refer to two aspects of consciousness. Meditation on tangible form is called *sākāra-dhyāna* (meditation on form). On the other hand, meditation on the imperceptible or intangible aspect is called *nirākāra-dhyāna* (meditation on the formless). To remain conscious during *nirākāra-dhyāna*, one should be properly prepared. In general, the mind is inclined toward the manifested objective reality. Before stepping onto the ground of *nirākāra-dhyāna*, it is advisable to focus on a point called *lakṣya*. There are three kinds of focus: gross (*sthūla*), medium (*madhyama*), and subtle (*sūkṣma*). A gross focus point (*sthūla-lakṣya*) is perceptible through the senses. This could be an image of the deities, a spiritual master, or great enlightened beings. Middle focus (*madhyama-lakṣya*) involves mental perception. It may be the *japa* or an inner visualization of the deities. Finally, subtle focus (*sūkṣma-lakṣya*) reflects on the *mahā-vākyas*, or "the great Vedantic sayings."

Sthūla-lakṣya

The mind must rely on an object to stabilize itself. Therefore, it is advisable to focus on the deities to begin the practice of *sthūla-lakṣya*. Observe the deities of Īśvara such as Śrī Śrī Rādhā Śyāmasundara, Jagannātha, Baladeva and Subhadrā, Śrī Śrī Kāliya Kṛṣṇa, or Lord Nṛsiṁhadeva. Pay attention to images or sculptures of enlightened beings like Jesus, Buddha, or Caitanya. If you are perceptive, you will see that it is possible to detect, to a greater or lesser extent, something of the unmanifested in each of them. When you find yourself in front of enlightened beings, you will see unmistakable traces of the transcendental in their gaze, in their words, and in their presence. You will be able to recognize the seed from the fruits and flowers of the tree.

We are all an expression of divine nature, but it flows more clearly through some beings. They not only know about That, but they practically are That and seem to speak to us from paradise itself. They are normal human beings, but not ordinary; they are regular individuals, but very different. Although they walk, talk, and move on the objective plane, they express the unmanifested. An intoxicating fragrance emanates from their presence and their silence sounds like a captivating melody. Worship and meditation in the physical proximity of such beings is said to benefit the meditator.

Undoubtedly, every human being is an expression of the Divine. However, the enlightened ones are divinity expressed as humanity. Whoever meditates on them and allows their presence to penetrate the heart will benefit eternally. In the depths of the soul, what is manifested will gradually fade away, while what is unmanifested will remain. If a disciple and a visitor are in the presence of an enlightened master, they will have completely different experiences. The visitor will only perceive the master's manifested human aspect, while the disciple will connect with the master's transcendental and unmanifested aspect. The visitor will not perceive the seed, but only see the objective form of the tree. The disciple and the visitor will not understand each other, because, although both speak of the same person, they are talking about completely different aspects.

Madhyama-lakṣya

Only those who have focused on Kṛṣṇa on the objective plane will be able to access the subjective perception of him.

1. *Vaidhi-sādhana*, or "external practice": The initial steps are *vaidhi-bhakti*, in the form of *pūjā*, ceremonies, and rituals.
2. *Antaraṅga-sādhana*, or "inner practice": Then comes *rāgānugā-bhakti*, consisting of *mānasa-pūjā*, or "mental worship."
3. *Nirākāra-sādhana,* or "formless practice": Finally, *svarūpa-smṛti*, or "remembrance of our true nature."

Likewise, those who repeat the *māhā-mantra* perceive magic in their chanting, a vestige of the Absolute and the transcendental. Thus, they will resonate with the words of Śrīla Rūpa Goswami:

तुण्डे ताण्डविनी रतिं वितनुते तुण्डावलीलब्धये
कर्णक्रोडकडम्बिनी घटयते कर्णार्बुदेभ्यः स्पृहाम् ।
चेतःप्राङ्गणसङ्गिनी विजयते सर्वेन्द्रियाणां कृतिं
नो जाने जनिता कियद्भिरमृतैः कृष्णेति वर्णद्वयी ॥

tuṇḍe tāṇḍavinī ratiṁ vitanute tuṇḍāvalī-labdhaye
karṇa-kroḍa-kaḍambinī ghaṭayate karṇārbudebhyaḥ spṛhām
cetaḥ-prāṅgaṇa-saṅginī vijayate sarvendriyāṇāṁ kṛtiṁ
no jāne janitā kiyadbhir amṛtaiḥ kṛṣṇeti varṇa-dvayī

> I do not know how much nectar the two syllables 'Kṛṣ-ṇa' have produced. When the holy name of Kṛṣṇa is chanted, it appears to dance in the mouth. We then desire many, many mouths. When that name goes into the ear canals, we desire many millions of ears. And when the holy name dances in the courtyard of the heart, it conquers the activities of the mind, and all the senses become inert.
>
> (*Vidagdha-mādhava*, 1.15)

Sūkṣma-lakṣya

Sūkṣma-lakṣya means to reflect on the *mahā-vākyas*. Although there are many *mahā-vākyas*, each Veda has one that is most important. They speak to the eternal unity of the individual with the Whole, or *ātmā* with Brahman. The highest states of consciousness are expressed by reflecting on the Vedantic maxims. The four *mahā-vākyas* are:

प्रज्ञानं ब्रह्म।

prajñānaṁ brahma

Consciousness is Brahman.

(*Aitareya Upanishad* of the *Rig Veda*, 3.3)

अयमात्मा ब्रह्म ।

ayam ātmā brahma.

This Self (or Ātman) is Brahman.
(*Māṇḍukya Upanishad* of the *Atharva Veda*, 1.2)

तत्त्वमसि ।

tat tvam asi

Thou art That.
(*Chāndogya Upanishad* of the *Sama Veda*, 6.8.7)

अहं ब्रह्मास्मि ।

ahaṁ brahmāsmi

I am Brahman.
(*Bṛhad-āraṇyaka Upanishad* of the *Yajur Veda*, 1.4.10)

"...worshippers of the unmanifested."

In *nirākāra-sādhana*, *nirākāra* concentration leads to dissolution, or *laya*. When practitioners relax, their minds sink like a stone in a lake. In this *laya* state, they lose both their inner and outer awareness, just as in deep sleep. There are those whose mental activity easily reduces. However, as thoughts diminish, they might simply fall asleep. In this case, although thought is abandoned, consciousness is also relinquished. When they are so attached to the thought process that their minds are part of who they are, stopping thought causes them to fall asleep. Reality is achieved only when they transcend thought without falling asleep. Unconsciousness leads only to sleep, not to reality. In such a situation, consciousness is immersed in unconsciousness. But in meditation, it is unconsciousness that submerges into consciousness.

To recognize an object, we observe its characteristics but not its essence. We notice its attributes and ignore its permanent and unchanging nature. However, some objects lack concrete manifestations. For example, numbers are just ideas. In the manifested dimension, we perceive events interwoven in a relationship of cause and effect. Even an abstract object such as an idea must have a cause, and sometimes the cause is a mere concept. It may be difficult to determine its cause, but it must exist. Similarly, for God to exist, even as an idea or concept, it must have a transcendental cause. *Asaṁbhūti* refers to such a transcendental cause, the unmanifested God. It is the origin of everything manifested. It is impossible to conceptualize or outline it, which would be incompatible with its causeless nature. And when we finally know, we know that we know, but we do not know how we know. We know that we always knew and that is all we need to know.

We are discussing the existence of the unique

unmanifested reality, unknown and unknowable to the human mind. This reality underlies all objects. It has been called *śūnyatā*, or "emptiness." St. John of the Cross referred to it in the opening verses of his poem "How well I know that fountain":

> How well I know that fountain's rushing flow
> Although by night
>
> Its deathless spring is hidden. Even so
> Full well I guess from whence its sources flow
> Though it be night.
>
> Its origin (since it has none) none knows:
> But that all origin from it arose
> Although by night.
>
> I know there is no other thing so fair
> And earth and heaven drink refreshment there
> Although by night
>
> Full well I know its depth no man can sound
> And that no ford to cross it can be found
> Though by night.

Unmanifested reality is the background of all things and all beings. Mentally, we conceptualize the unmanifested as a nothingness devoid of content. However, reality transcends the limited possibilities of our mind. Reality, or emptiness, resides in all beings, including our own being. The manifested is much more than just an emanation from the unmanifested; it is a school of self-knowledge. If the manifested were only an emanation, the product of a simple casual explosion, it would be like a sculpture emerging from the hands of a sculptor. But the manifested is not a static object; it has life and yearns to know and rejoin its sculptor. This longing is an essential part of the manifested, because the piece was sculpted from the only raw material that the artist had available: himself. The manifested sculpture was made from the sculptor's own body and soul. Therefore, it yearns to be reunited with itself.

On the manifested plane, feelings of estrangement, alienation, or separation from the origin reign. The human need to return to their origin causes them profound discomfort and anguish. They suffer deep longings for the original source and harbor nostalgia for absolute peace and love. This has been the drive of every seeker of Truth for generations. Those who attain ultimate reality only discover that such a separation never really existed. However, these words have no value without direct experience. Though the words of one who has attained the reality of the soul may be helpful, they will never be enough. Nothing in this world can substitute for directly perceiving Truth.

"Those who worship the manifested enter the region of darkness; even worse happens to the worshippers of the unmanifested."

Observation allows us to clearly perceive the simultaneous unity and difference between the manifested and the unmanifested. Many consider our body to be part of the very basis of manifested reality. However, if we observe closely, we realize that the body is nothing more than a collection of images, sensations, and perceptions that appear in the mind. Instead of being a solid object, the manifested body is merely a mental image. Everything we know about it comes from this mental image and the sensations that appear in our mind.

Recent scientific experiments have begun to demonstrate that matter is not as solid as we once thought. What has been called matter is not matter, but energy with a vibration so low it is barely perceptible. Matter is not solid, but is consciousness reduced to a perceptible point. The finite mind is a contraction and localization of infinite consciousness. Clearly, unmanifested consciousness cannot know a finite object. If it could, the existence of the finite object would threaten the infinitude of unmanifested consciousness.

During deep sleep, perception of the manifested world is completely gone. Unmanifested consciousness is experienced, devoid of content. Consciousness turns inward and relinquishes all connection with mind and body. In such a state, consciousness relaxes and knows only itself. The only way for unmanifested consciousness to perceive a finite and manifested object is by ignoring its infinite nature and becoming a finite mind. Unmanifested consciousness can only perceive the manifested universe by becoming a finite manifested mind itself.

When we sleep, the dream world can be perceived only from the perspective of the dream. If you dream that you are walking around New Delhi, you will be one of the people present in your dream and you will experience the city from the perspective of the dream experience. Consciousness can only perceive the dream by situating itself as a character in the dream. Therefore, in order to perceive the finite universe, infinite consciousness must rely on the finite manifested mind. For this purpose, there is a process of simultaneous creation and identification with form, which results in the finite mind.

In order to perceive a manifested object, the unmanifested consciousness must limit itself and become a manifested subject-form. Unmanifested consciousness perceives the manifested world from the perspective of the manifested form or body. However, in order to know itself, by itself, and in itself, consciousness does not need to transform itself into a finite mind. Just as infinite and unmanifested consciousness cannot perceive a finite and manifested object, the finite and manifested mind cannot access infinite and unmanifested consciousness.

In order to perceive objective reality, consciousness

reduces its vision in order to become embodied. Doing this allows it to know the manifested reality from the perspective of a particular body. Self-knowledge is a path of involution that involves relaxing the focus of attention and divesting all limitations. To become self-aware, consciousness simply ceases to identify with the finite form and mind. Death is dispersing consciousness from a particular location. But when the release of such a contraction occurs, consciousness does not dissolve.

An embodied person is like a whirlpool in the sea, and the unmanifested consciousness is like water. At death, the whirlpool dissolves, but nothing really disappears because everything is water. The water remains devoid of a form and a mind. The body–mind complex is nothing more than a whirlpool in the sea; it is a localization of consciousness where manifested reality appears. With death, this whirlpool disperses, and its contents remain as consciousness. Elements of previously dispersed content can return to form new locations and finite minds. The residues of a previous finite mind can form a new whirlpool. This is what we call reincarnation.

देहिनोऽस्मिन्यथा देहे कौमारं यौवनं जरा ।
तथा देहान्तरप्राप्तिर्धीरस्तत्र न मुह्यति ॥

dehino 'smin yathā dehe
kaumāraṁ yauvanaṁ jarā
tathā dehāntara-prāptir
dhīras tatra na muhyati

> As the embodied soul continuously passes, in this body, from boyhood to youth to old age, the soul similarly passes into another body at death. A sober person is not bewildered by such a change.
> (Bhagavad Gita, 2.13)

Reincarnation is often misunderstood as a change of physical body. However, material bodies do not become embodied just because they are different accumulations of sensations, images, and perceptions. Childhood, adolescence, youth, and adulthood are nothing more than different images, perceptions, and sensations. Therefore, reincarnation is a phenomenon at the consciousness level.

What we call material bodies are appearances in the finite mind. Consciousness contracts and becomes a finite mind, appearing as a form and a world. With relaxation, consciousness abandons the mind and the body. Then, the manifested universe of names and forms disappears. Contraction and relaxation alternate, as pulsations of a single consciousness: contraction and distention, localization and dispersion, being and non-being, on and off, manifestation and non-manifestation.

Hinduism accepts that existence moves in eternal circles of creation, preservation, and dissolution. Even each of these cosmic states, or pulsations, is governed by its own deity. Brahma creates, Viṣṇu maintains, and Śiva dissolves. The manifested and unmanifested are not different realities, but two states of the same consciousness. At the end of the path, we arrive at the realization that the essence of the manifested and unmanifested is exactly the same and that the primordial substance we seek is the same as the seeker.

Mantra 13

अन्यदेवाहुः सम्भवादन्यदाहुरसम्भवात् ।
इति शुश्रुम धीराणां ये नस्तद्विचचक्षिरे ॥

anyad evāhuḥ sambhavād
anyad āhur asambhavāt
iti śuśruma dhīrāṇāṁ
ye nas tad vicacakṣire

It is stated that different results are obtained from the manifested and the unmanifested. All this has been heard from the lips of the sages, who have imparted it to us.

Commentary:

We face two different directions, each leading to a different result. We obtain certain benefits by devoting ourselves to the manifested and others if we consecrate ourselves to the unmanifested. Each one also has its disadvantages.

Cultivating the manifested leads to progress in different areas in our society, from medicine to communications, nuclear weapons to interplanetary travel, and architecture to engineering. The great discoveries and advances of humankind originate in our effort to conquer nature and overcome the environment, which is clearly very important for society. However, without a parallel development of consciousness, scientific and technological progress can cause harm, pain, misfortune, and misery.

In other words, growth in the realm of the manifested and the relative without a corresponding evolution in the level of consciousness can bring disaster. An electric saw is very useful, but in the hands of an ape it is very dangerous. We can also observe this imbalance at the individual level. For example, there are those who perform intense physical exercise and neglect their inner world. They develop muscle mass but are spiritually starved. Others accumulate wealth in dollars and diamonds, but they suffer from a true destitution of the soul: wealth in the wallet but poverty in the spirit.

On the other hand, exclusively worshipping the unmanifested as something separate from the manifested can lead to contempt for the world, and this resembles darkness. Many aspirants to the Absolute despise and even lacerate their body in the name of holiness, but they do not understand the body's importance in the evolution of the soul.

Attaching oneself to the unmanifested, as something separate from the manifested, leads to contempt for the world and rejection of the body. But if we wish to evolve, we should live deeply. Otherwise, our development will be only horizontal, and we will grow sideways toward the extremes. Without growing roots in the depths of existence, we will become extremists. It is essential that we evolve inward and anchor ourselves in life.

It would be a mistake to go after either only the manifested or the unmanifested. Clinging to just one of these would be like escaping from one state to end up at its opposite. All extremism represents a kind of darkness. Going after only the manifested will keep us within *saṁsāra*, or "the circle of repeated births and deaths," as slaves of the pleasures of the body. But if we strive only for the unmanifested, we may succeed in dissolving ourselves indiscriminately, but without any kind of transcendence.

As we fall asleep, we disappear into a state of unconsciousness and upon awakening, we are reborn into a new day. But sleeping is not consciously transcending the manifested; it is just choosing its opposite. If we choose the unmanifested as the opposite of the manifested, we will not transcend the relative duality, but reaffirm it. The door to transcendence is not escape but observation and meditation.

The death of the egoic phenomenon refers to the transcendental state in which consciousness is recognized. Different religions and spiritual paths use the term "mystical death." The Jewish Talmud calls this as *mitat neshikah*, or "the kiss of death" in Hebrew. In Sufism, "dying before death" is a conscious and voluntary death prior to physical passing. It occurs when we transcend our concepts of manifestation and non-manifestation. It means discovering that life and death are illusory ideas that obscure the simple reality that we are, always were, and always will be.

An ancient teaching in Zen Buddhism says "if dharma is practiced during the day, one can die in peace at nightfall." The day represents our activity on the manifested plane, while nightfall is our experience of extinction, or the unmanifested. The same consciousness assumes two apparently different states; therefore, only if our daily activity is total, so will be the inactivity at nightfall. If we live intensely present every instant of our life, every evening we can experience that it is a perfect night to die. As the Buddha said: "Those who are attentive in the present will never die; for those who do not pay attention to the present moment, it is as if they are already dead."

When we close our eyes and lie calmly in bed, our bodily and mental activity decreases. However, many of us find it extremely difficult to close our eyes in peace and tranquility. During the day, we feel restless, anxious, impatient, and agitated. We are not where we are and our mind constantly wanders. We are never really present in mind, soul, and body in what we do.

Zen is an immensely wise and simple way of realization. It recommends that we live in the moment of life and we die at the moment of death. Living refers to being with the totality of who we are, as manifested entities, fully surrendering our minds and bodies and being immersed in the present task. At nightfall, we retire to rest. Along with our surrender to rest in the unmanifested, the manifested world of names and forms dies.

If we are prepared to die, we are prepared to live; if we accept the unmanifest, we can act within the manifest. Our activity in the manifested must always be rooted in the unmanifested. This means acting from peace and moving from silence. From the perspective of death, life acquires a new meaning. From the unmanifested, the manifested becomes magical and fresh.

"All this has been heard from the lips of the sages, who have imparted it to us."

In this mantra, we see the spirit of the disciple, who attributes all wisdom to the grace of the master. From the disciples' perspective, the wisdom they share flows directly from the lips of their master. If someone benefits, they attribute it to their guru. Disciples consider themselves to be the work of their master.

It is difficult to define the mysterious phenomenon of

discipleship. In the Western world, people often confuse disciples and masters for students and teachers. This is a serious mistake, because these two relationships are completely different. The foundations of the teacher–student relationship are instruction, information, and knowledge. On the other hand, the master–disciple relationship is based on silence, meditation, and wisdom. The student studies; the disciple learns. Studying means memorizing a certain subject that will later be used for academic purposes. Often the student studies just to pass exams. Studying means storing information in a corner of the mind. Learning means digesting wisdom, making it part of ourselves, and applying it to our daily life. We do not know the wisdom we learn; we become this wisdom.

You could place students in front of Jesus, Buddha, or Lao Tzu, but they will not recognize the master. They will only see a teacher. Students cannot have a connection with a master if they are loaded with concepts, beliefs, and conclusions. Discipleship means being predisposed to acquire wisdom, which requires setting aside all preconceived ideas.

तद्विद्धि प्रणिपातेन परिप्रश्नेन सेवया ।
उपदेक्ष्यन्ति ते ज्ञानं ज्ञानिनस्तत्त्वदर्शिनः ॥

tad viddhi praṇipātena
paripraśnena sevayā
upadekṣyanti te jñānaṁ
jñāninas tattva-darśinaḥ

> Just try to learn the Truth by approaching a spiritual master. Inquire from him submissively and render service unto him. Self-realized souls can impart knowledge unto you because they have seen the Truth.
>
> (Bhagavad Gita, 4.34)

To approach a *tattva-darśinaḥ*, it is essential to be a disciple, because students cannot connect with a master. They may get closer physically, but there will never be a real encounter between the two.

> जननमरणादिसंसारनलसन्तप्तो दीप्तशिरा जलराशिमिव उपहारपानिः श्रोत्रियं ब्रह्मनिष्ठंगुरुमुपसृत्य तमनुसरति ॥
>
> *janana-maraṇādi-saṁsāra-nala-santapto dīpta-śirā jala-rāśim iva upahāra-pāniḥ śrotriyaṁ brahma-niṣṭhaṁ gurum upasṛtya tam anusarati.*
>
> Just as a person whose head is on fire runs to water, one burning from the fire of material existence—birth, death, old age, and disease—must run to a guru for relief. The guru must be fixed in the absolute Truth and well-versed in the scriptures. One should approach the guru with all that is needed to sacrifice, submit, and carry out the guru's instructions.
>
> (*Śrī Gauḍīya Kaṇṭha-hāra*, *Guru-tattva*, 1.6)

The phenomenon of the spiritual master will always be a puzzle for rational students. For students, what matters are the words and the teachings of the teacher. For disciples, what is essential is the master. The disciple sees no difference between the master and the teachings. The master is the way and the Truth. It is enough to remain silent in the presence of the master because silence is the message and the answer. In the presence of the master, there are no questions or doubts.

Someday, students will become teachers and recite the same information to the new students. However, all the knowledge will be recycled. Perhaps they will even talk about religion. But without having experienced what religion is, they will only talk about theology and mythology. Perhaps they will be able to lecture about God, but without having experienced God, this will be second-hand knowledge. If nothing divine has touched their heart, they will tell stories about what happened to some saint thousands of years ago. Perhaps they will write books about love without ever having loved anyone, not even themselves.

Teachers declaims ideas, concepts, explanations, and arguments without having any clue about the Truth. Students hear about scriptures, philosophies, theologies, and ideologies, but nothing about the Truth. Disciples are not interested in hearing words about anything, but in being that which is spoken of. Students hear the teacher's words; disciples listen to the master. Hearing a teacher and listening to a master are two diametrically opposed processes. Hearing the words of a master changes the periphery, but the inner self remains exactly the same. Listening to a master does not add information; it brings about transformation.

Students desire to know the Truth while disciples aspire to be the Truth; this is the main difference between them. For disciples, the words *about God* are far removed from God; the words *about Truth* are light years away from *Truth. About* is not knowledge of anything, but only a layer of lacquer covering ignorance. The approach of students is to acquire, obtain, reach, take, accumulate, buy, appropriate, seize, grab, hoard, and possess. Students are greedy because their efforts are aimed at seizing the wealth of knowledge. On the other hand, the spirit of disciples is to experience, feel, notice, perceive, distinguish, observe, watch, see, examine, investigate, and explore. Discipleship is free of greed and jealousy, since its intention is not to obtain or seize something, but to experience oneself in reality.

The master–disciple relationship also differs from the leader–follower relationship. Disciples are not followers. Followers are like pendulums that can swing from fanaticism to enmity. Those who are able to follow leaders blindly can also hate them. The leader–follower relationship is neither religious nor spiritual, but political.

While followers blindly fall in line behind leaders, disciples try to understand their masters. Follower bond with leaders through fanatical attachment, while disciples do so through love and devotion. Attachment is a mere mental phenomenon. Masters and disciples do not meet in the mind, but in the heart. Their loving relationship is the highest that exists since it transcends body and mind. However, for those who associate love with romantic soap operas, this relationship is incomprehensible. We idealize the love between Romeo and Juliet, but true love is that between Moses and Joshua, Arjuna and Kṛṣṇa, Rabbi Nachman and Rabbi Nathan, and Jesus and Mary Magdalene.

A life centered on our own needs and whims leads to suffering. If our sole purpose is to satisfy our ego's demands, we are doomed to frustration. As we become aware of the suffering that the egoic phenomenon entails, we look for ways to transcend it. The master is the hook where we can simply hang our ego.

तद्विज्ञानार्थं स गुरुमेवाभिगच्छेत्समित्पाणिः श्रोत्रियं ब्रह्मनिष्ठम् ॥

tad vijñānārthaṁ sa gurum evābhigacchet samit-pāṇiḥ śrotriyaṁ brahma-niṣṭham.

In order to learn transcendental science, one must approach a bona fide spiritual master in disciplic succession, who is fixed in the absolute Truth.

(*Muṇḍaka Upanishad*, 1.2.12)

यस्य देवे परा भक्तिः यथा देवे तथा गुरौ ।
तस्यैते कथिता ह्यर्थाः प्रकाशन्ते महात्मनः ॥

yasya deve parā bhaktir
yathā deve tathā gurau
tasyaite kathaitā hy arthāḥ
prakaśante mahātmanaḥ

> The importance of the Vedas is only fully revealed to those great souls who serve a guru and the Divine with implicit faith.
> (*Śvetāśvatara Upanishad*, 6.23)

Love is the basis of discipleship. Without love, surrender will not be genuine. Disciples' love must be so authentic that the master will be the center of their lives. They abandon everything for their guru. They renounce all their defenses until they reach the point of maximum vulnerability. Upon reaching unconditional love and total surrender, the master–disciple fusion takes place. Only in loving surrender, disciples melt like salt dolls in the ocean of the master and they become nobody. Their surrender is like dying, because from that moment on, the master lives through them. Disciples become the shadow of one who is no one, that is, the shadow of someone who is the Whole manifested in a form. And that is only the beginning, because it will be followed by surrender to the unmanifested. Like a river flowing into the sea, disciples flow into the master. Like a silkworm, disciples die at the feet of the master to be reborn as butterflies. If a sincere desire to transcend yourself awakens deep within you, trust that existence will place a master on your path.

Mantra 14

सम्भूतिं च विनाशं च यस्तद्वेदोभयꣳसह ।
विनाशेन मृत्युं तीर्त्वा सम्भूत्याऽमृतमश्नुते ॥

sambhūtiṁ ca vināśaṁ ca
yas tad vedobhayaṁ saha
vināśena mṛtyuṁ tīrtvā
sambhūty-āmṛtam aśnute

One who worships God in his personal and impersonal aspects simultaneously transcends death through the worship of the manifested and realizes immortality through the worship of the unmanifested.

Commentary:

Because we think we are separate entities residing within solid bodies, we experience an apparent duality of two realities, manifested and unmanifested. The manifested is empirical and the unmanifested is subjective. We believe that an observer resides inside our body and observes a separate universe through the senses. Such a conclusion is based on the idea that there is an entity called "I" that lives within a solid structure and experiences a diversity of names and forms different from itself. Thus, a fractured reality is experienced, which is divided into observer and observed, subject and object, unmanifested and manifested.

This text brings up the ancient controversy between the objective and subjective paths, that is, manifested and unmanifested divinity. This is the eternal debate between the devotional and intellectual paths, or *bhakti* and *jñāna*. The manifested God is the creator of the universe who participates in the pastimes of different religions. This personal God has attributes and qualities, like Īśvara or Bhagavān. This is the God who liberated the people of Israel from slavery in Egypt and the Father Jesus prayed to. The sage Parāśara Muni Bhagavān believes God is the sole possessor of total beauty, wealth, fame, strength, knowledge, and renunciation. It is the aspect of God that atheists resist the most and is the center of countless controversies. On the other hand, the God of the unmanifested is the inconceivable and indescribable Absolute. If we have understood this triad of mantras, we know that the heart and the intellect, far from being contradictory, complement each other. Both share the same goal of caressing and knowing the ultimate Truth.

However, we are not talking about information but existential knowledge. For *bhaktas*, such knowledge is only possible when loving; for *jñānīs*, knowing means becoming what is known. For *bhaktas*, loving is synonymous with knowing. Intimate knowledge is only possible through love; therefore, love, in its most refined expression, will be sought after first. For *jñānīs*, it is impossible to love without really knowing.

The Bible uses the Hebrew term *yada*, or "knew", to describe the most intimate connection between the first human beings who were created: *Adam yada et hava*, that is, "Adam knew Eve." The same word is used to describe knowledge of God: *ve'yadata hayom va'hashevota el levabecha*, or "and you shall know this day and return to your heart." Kṛṣṇadāsa Kavirāja Gosvāmī expresses the same idea:

অনর্পিতচরীং চিরাৎ করুণয়াবতীর্ণঃ কলৌ
সমর্পয়িতুমুন্নতোজ্জ্বলরসাং স্বভক্তিশ্রিয়ম্ ।
হরিঃ পুরটসুন্দরদ্যুতিকদম্বসন্দীপিতঃ
সদা হৃদয়কন্দরে স্ফুরতু বঃ শচীনন্দনঃ ॥

anarpita-carīṁ cirāt karuṇayāvatīrṇaḥ kalua
samarpayitum unnatojjvala-rasāṁ sva-bhakti-śriyam
hariḥ puraṭa-sundara-dyuti-kadamba-sandīpitaḥ
sadā hṛdaya-kandare sphuratu vaḥ śacī-nandanaḥ

> May the Supreme Lord, who is known as the son of Śrīmatī Śacī-devī, be transcendentally situated in the innermost core of your heart. Resplendent with the radiance of molten gold, He has descended in the Age of Kali by His causeless mercy to bestow what no incarnation has ever offered before: the most elevated mellow of devotional service, the mellow of conjugal love.
> (*Śrī Caitanya-caritāmṛta*, "*Ādi-līlā*," 3.4).

Clearly, conjugal love comes with the most intimate knowledge of the beloved.

The Torah states:

> וְאָהַבְתָּ אֵת ה' אֱלֹקֶיךָ בְּכָל לְבָבְךָ וּבְכָל נַפְשְׁךָ וּבְכָל מְאֹדֶךָ.
> (דברים ו', ה')

> *ve'ahavta et hashem elokeicha be'chol levavcha u've'chol nafshecha u've'chol me'odecha.*

> And you shall love the Lord your God with all your heart and with all your soul and with all your might.
> (Deuteronomy, 6:5)

Sages along the history commented on this phrase of the Torah. The following are a handful of these commentaries:

Rabbi Avraham Ibn Ezra says:

"בְּכָל לְבָבְךָ וּבְכָל נַפְשֶׁךָ" - הַלֵּב הוּא הַדַּעַת, וְהוּא כִּנּוּי לָרוּחַ הַמַּשְׂכֶּלֶת, כִּי הוּא הַמַּרְכֶּבֶת הָרִאשׁוֹנָה; וְכֵן "חֲכַם לֵב" (שמות ל"א, ו'); "קוֹנֶה לֵב" (משלי ט"ו, ל"ב).
(פירוש רבי אברהם אבן עזרא על התורה, דברים ו', ה')

"With all thy heart, and with all thy soul." *B'chol levavcha u'v'chol nafshecha.* The heart refers to knowledge, denoting the spirit of intelligence (the rational soul), for the heart is its first vehicle. The same is expressed in the verses "wise-hearted" (Exodus, 36:1) and "He who acquired a heart (i.e. wisdom)" (Proverbs, 19:8).

Ramban, Rabbi Moshe Ben Nachman says:

"בְּכָל לְבָבְךָ"- עַל דַּעַת הַמִּדְרָשׁ (ספרי ואתחנן, ו') הַלֵּב הַנִּזְכָּר כָּאן הוּא הַכֹּחַ הַמִּתְאַוֶּה, כְּעִנְיַן "תַּאֲוַת לִבּוֹ נָתַתָּ לּוֹ" (תהלים כ"א, ג') "אַל תַּחְמֹד יָפְיָהּ בִּלְבָבֶךָ" (משלי ו', כ"ה) אִם כֵּן, "בְּכָל נַפְשְׁךָ"- הַנֶּפֶשׁ הַמַּשְׂכֶּלֶת...

ור"א אָמַר כִּי "נַפְשְׁךָ"- הַמִּתְאַוָּה. כְּמוֹ "כְּנַפְשְׁךָ שָׂבְעֶךָ" (דברים כ"ג, כ"ה), "נֶפֶשׁ שְׂבֵעָה תָּבוּס נֹפֶת" (משלי כ"ז, ז'), "אַל תִּתְּנֵנִי בְּנֶפֶשׁ צָרָי" (תהלים כ"ז, י"ב). "וּבְכָל לְבָבְךָ" הוּא הַדַּעַת, וְהוּא כִּנּוּי לָרוּחַ הַמַּשְׂכֶּלֶת, כִּי הִיא הַמֶּרְכָּבָה הָרִאשׁוֹנָה לוֹ, וְכָמוֹהוּ "חֲכַם לֵב יִקַּח מִצְוֹת" (משלי י', ח'). וּדְבָרוֹ קָרוֹב בְּפֵרוּשׁ "בְּכָל לְבָבְךָ", מִמָּה שֶׁאָמַר "וְהָיוּ הַדְּבָרִים הָאֵלֶּה וְגוֹ' עַל לְבָבֶךָ".

וְטַעַם "וּבְכָל מְאֹדֶךָ" כְּלוֹמַר: מְאֹד מְאֹד וְהַטַּעַם: רַב רַב אֱהֹב אוֹתוֹ. וְעַל דַּעַת רַבּוֹתֵינוּ (ברכות נ"ד, א') "בְּכָל מָמוֹנְךָ" וְיִקָּרֵא הַמָּמוֹן "מְאֹד" כִּי יְכֻנֶּה אוֹתוֹ בְּרִבּוּי כְּמוֹ שֶׁקּוֹרֵא לוֹ "הָמוֹן": "טוֹב מְעַט לַצַּדִּיק מֵהֲמוֹן רְשָׁעִים רַבִּים" (תהלים ל"ז, ט"ז) "וְהִנָּם כְּכָל הֲמוֹן יִשְׂרָאֵל" (מלכים ב' ז', י"ג)...

(רמב"ן על התורה, דברים ו', ה')

"With all your heart." According to *Midrash Sifre*, (*Va'etchanan*, 6); the heart which is mentioned here is the power of desire, as in the following: "You have granted him his heart's desire" (Psalms, 21:3); "lust not after her beauty in thy heart." (Proverbs, 6:25). And therefore, "with all thy soul" denotes the intellectual [capacity rather than the sensual capacity of the] soul…

But Rabbi Eliezer (in the same *midrash*) holds the opposite: that "With all your soul" denotes the power of desire, as it is said: "Until your soul is satisfied" (Deuteronomy, 23:25), "A sated soul disdains honey" (Proverbs, 27:7), and "Do not subject me to the will (lit. 'soul') of my foes" (Psalms, 27:12), And "with all your heart" is the knowledge, and is denoting the intellectual soul, for the heart is its first vehicle, and this is supported in the verse "He whose heart is wise accepts commands" (Proverbs, 10:8).

And the meaning of "With all your might" is "very very much". Means, love him a lot. And according to our Rabbis (*Berachot*, 54) "With all your might" is the wealth, and the wealth is called 'very much' because it is called after its quantity...

Ralbag, Rabbi Levi Ben Gershom, says:

"בְּכָל לְבָבְךָ"- יָדוּעַ כִּי הַלֵּב יֵאָמֵר עַל הָרָצוֹן, וְהִנֵּה בָּאָדָם שְׁנֵי מִינִים מֵהָרָצוֹן וְהַחֵפֶץ; הָאֶחָד הוּא הַכֹּחַ הַמִּתְעוֹרֵר שֶׁהוּא נִמְשָׁךְ לְצִיּוּר הַדִּמְיוֹן, וְהַשֵּׁנִי הוּא הַכֹּחַ הַמִּתְעוֹרֵר שֶׁהוּא נִמְשָׁךְ לְצִיּוּר הַשֵּׂכֶל. וּכְבָר יִרְאֶה הָאָדָם בְּעַצְמוֹ לִפְעָמִים שְׁנֵי אֵלּוּ הַכֹּחוֹת יַחַד, וְיַחֲלֹק זֶה עַל זֶה. וּבָרָעִים יִגְבַּר הַיֵּצֶר הָרַע וּבַטּוֹבִים יְנַצֵּחַ הַיֵּצֶר הַטּוֹב. וּכְאִלּוּ הִזְהִיר בָּזֶה, וְצִוָּה שֶׁיַּכְנִיעַ הָאָדָם כָּל מִינֵי רְצוֹנוֹ לְאַהֲבַת הַשֵּׁם יִתְעַלֶּה; וְיִמָּשֵׁךְ מֵהָאַהֲבָה הַזֹּאת שֶׁיִּשְׁמֹר מִצְוֹתָיו, כִּי הָאוֹהֵב יִשְׁתַּדֵּל לַעֲשׂוֹת רְצוֹן אוֹהֲבוֹ כְּפִי הַיְּכֹלֶת.

"With all your heart." It is known that the word "heart" indicates the power of will, and in the human being we encounter two types of will: The first is the awakening power which is attracted to the forms drawn by the imagination, and the second is the awakening power which is attracted to the forms of the intellect. One may observe in oneself these two powers opposing one another. In bad (people), the bad inclination will overpower, and in good (people), the good inclination will conquer. And seems that (The Divine) warned and guided us here, that a man should surrender both types of his will power to the love of the Divine Lord. As a result of this love, he will be attracted to keep the Lord's *precepts*, because the lover would always try to do the will of his loved one as much as he can.

"**וְאָהַבְתָּ אֵת ה' אֱלֹקֶיךָ**"- צִוָּנוּ בְּזֶה הַמַּאֲמָר לֶאֱהֹב הַשֵּׁם יִתְעַלֶּה. וּלְפִי שֶׁהָאַהֲבָה, מְבֹאָר מֵעִנְיָנָהּ שֶׁלֹּא תִּהְיֶה לְדָבָר שֶׁאֵין לָנוּ בּוֹ שׁוּם הַשָּׂגָה, כָּל שֶׁכֵּן כְּשֶׁלֹּא תִּהְיֶה בְּזֶה הָאֹפֶן הַשָּׁלֵם אֲשֶׁר זָכַר פֹּה, הִנֵּה יְחַיֵּב זֶה הַצִּוּוּי, שֶׁנַּעֲשֶׂה בְּדֶרֶךְ שֶׁתִּהְיֶה לָנוּ הַשָּׂגָה מָה בְּזֶה הַשֵּׁם הַנִּכְבָּד, כְּדֵי שֶׁנִּתְעוֹרֵר מִפְּנֵי זֶה לְאַהֲבוֹ; וְכָל מָה שֶׁנּוֹסִיף הַשָּׂגָה בּוֹ יִתְעַלֶּה, נוֹסִיף לְאַהֲבָה אוֹתוֹ. וְהִנֵּה זֶה יֻשַּׂג לָנוּ מִצַּד שָׁקְדֵנוּ עַל מִצְוֹת הַתּוֹרָה, כִּי הֵם יְיַשִּׁירוּנוּ אֶל הַשָּׂגָתוֹ יִתְעַלֶּה, כְּמוֹ שֶׁבֵּאַרְנוּ בְּזֶה הַסֵּפֶר, וּמִצַּד הַחֲקִירָה עַל פְּעֻלּוֹת הַשֵּׁם יִתְעַלֶּה הַנִּפְלָאוֹת הַמֻּשָּׂגוֹת לָנוּ מֵעִנְיַן אֵלּוּ הַנִּמְצָאוֹת אֲשֶׁר אֶצְלֵנוּ. וְהוּא מְבֹאָר, כִּי כְּשֶׁיַּעֲמֹד הָאָדָם עַל זֶה, תִּהְיֶה אַהֲבָתוֹ הַשֵּׁם יִתְעַלֶּה הַיּוֹתֵר חֲזָקָה שֶׁבְּכָל הָאַהֲבוֹת אֲשֶׁר אֶצְלוֹ, כִּי סִבּוֹת הָאַהֲבָה הֵם הַשְּׁלֵמוּת וְהַמַּעֲלָה וְהָעַרְבוּת וְהַתּוֹעֶלֶת, כְּמוֹ שֶׁנִּזְכַּר בְּסֵפֶר הַמִּדּוֹת. וּלְפִי שֶׁהַשֵּׁם יִתְעַלֶּה הוּא בְּתַכְלִית הַשְּׁלֵמוּת וְהַמַּעֲלָה, עַד שֶׁשְּׁלֵמוּת כָּל נִמְצָא זוּלָתוֹ - חִסָּרוֹן בְּיַחַס אֶל שְׁלֵמוּתוֹ יִתְעַלֶּה, הִנֵּה יִהְיֶה הַיּוֹתֵר נֶאֱהָב לְאֵין שִׁעוּר מִזֶּה הַצַּד.

(רלב"ג על התורה, דברים ו', ה')

"And you shall love the Lord your God." In this statement we were instructed to love the Divine Lord.

And because love, by its nature, cannot be directed to something that we completely cannot

> comprehend, and moreover, such love (to the incomprehensible) cannot be as complete, as it is required here (in our verse), therefore, this implies that we have to act in such a way that will provide a slight understanding of the blessed Lord, so that we will awaken to love Him. We find that this can be achieved through a serious effort to keep the precepts [mitzvot] of the Torah, because they will direct us to knowing Him, blessed be He, as we explained in this book, and through investigation of those wonderous, unknowable actions of the Divine Lord that are knowable for us in some way from our own reality. And it is explained, that when a will achieve this, his love for the Divine Lord will grow greater than any other of his loves. Because, as mentioned (in Aristotle's 'Book of Ethics' Book 8, Chapter 8): the causes of love are: excellence and completeness, superiority, pleasure, and benefit. And because the Divine Lord's excellence and superiority is so absolute and complete, in comparison to Him, any other completeness is incomplete, therefore, He is loved without measure.

The New Testament quotes this verse from the Torah and defines it as the main commandment. Both scriptures advise us to embrace the heart (*bhakti*) and mind (*jñāna*) simultaneously.

> Love the Lord your God with all your heart and with all your soul and with all your mind and with all your strength.
>
> (New Testament, Mark, 12:30)

While loving and knowing are not different, knowing is the fruit of love. Through *bhakti*, death is overcome, because to love is to die a little. And those who have loved know that there is life after dying of love – life in abundance. Through *jñāna*, you know that you are the only thing you can be.

"...transcends death through the worship of the manifested and realizes immortality through the worship of the unmanifested."

If I had to summarize all my teachings in one word, I would certainly choose *observation*. Observation without the mind's intervention places us face-to-face with naked reality, like the child in the story "The Emperor's New Clothes" by the Danish author Hans Christian Andersen. The story shows that what the public thinks is not necessarily true. Observation strips us of any kind of conditioning, which brings out our authenticity. What is apparent and false falls away and what is authentic and real remains. By observing empirical reality, we conclude that we are not the objects we perceive. While they come and go, we remain. Likewise, by observing the body, the breath, the mind, and the emotions, we also notice that we are none of these. Observation is the master key that allows us to open the doors of life and access the mystery.

Too many human beings live in ignorance, without even knowing what they do not know. Based on their own interpretation of reality, they identify themselves with their bodies and believe they are Americans, Hindus, Chileans, or Brazilians. They identify with the mind and define themselves as communists, Zionists, capitalists, rightists, or leftists. From our illusion, we believe we are a body and a mind observing a universe of solid objects. However, by carefully contemplating the manifested and its objective diversity, we will see that the experience of the empirical universe is only perception. What we believe is our physical body is a mere set of sensations, and the mind, a stream of thoughts. Obviously, neither sensations nor thoughts can perceive what is manifested. They are not part of the observing subject but belong to the manifested platform, that is, the world of the observed. Both the body and the mind are integral parts of what is perceived. That which observes or perceives is completely devoid of qualities, objective attributes, or dimensions; otherwise, it would be another observable object. It is important to understand that if perception had qualities and dimensions, it would be part of the manifested perceptible reality instead of being the witness or subject.

The perceiver is not absent even for a moment. It is always present and conscious of every experience. Although it is the foundation of all experience, it goes completely unnoticed because it lacks qualities. It did not even begin to exist at some point in time. However, we ignore it or overlook it due to its complete lack of attributes and dimensions. By identifying ourselves with the body and mind, we believe ourselves to be the witnesses of what is manifested or observed. Even from a relative reality, we refer to consciousness as the observer of the manifested. We consider ourselves to be witnesses of the body, the mind, and the universe of names and forms. Therefore, at this level of observation, the dualities of subject–object and observer–observed prevail. That which observes and knows is usually baptized with the name "I." The idea that a witness exists is an *upādhi*, or "conditioning," that is projected onto consciousness when we think we are a witness who is separate and different from what is observed.

Little by little, through observation, we approach the ultimate reality. At a certain point in our development, it is essential to awaken to the existence of that which resides with complete presence and awareness in the foundation of all experience. It is what recognizes any objective experience without being an object within it. It is not an object, because it completely lacks objective dimensions or attributes. It must be present and exist for any object to be perceived or experienced on the manifested plane. That is, consciousness is the background of objective experience. Our authentic nature is the conscious presence that perceives and illuminates manifested objectivity. When we ask ourselves whether we exist, the affirmative answer does not come from thought; it originates in the conscious recognition of consciousness itself. If we continue inquiring along these lines, we will not find any limitation or dependence on anything or anyone outside consciousness itself. In the same way that it knows it exists, it also knows it lacks any limits in time or space. It is clear that such testimony can only come from consciousness itself.

The reality of consciousness is often unnoticed because of misidentifications with thoughts, emotions, the body, or the mind. Misidentifications prevent us from perceiving perception or being aware of consciousness itself. By overlooking consciousness, we believe that manifested reality unfolds before consciousness and is completely different from it. However, looking closely at empirical experience shows us that it is impossible to demarcate the beginning of the observed object and the end of the conscious observer. The boundaries between subject and object in experience are not real. When listening to a melody, it is difficult to establish the end of the conscious listener and the beginning of the melody. There are no clear boundaries between us as observers and the universe of objective experience.

Even while dreaming, we experience a dual world of subject–object, although every person, animal, or thing exists only in us. However, upon awakening, it becomes obvious that the people in the dream, along with the space where everything appeared, all came is part of us. Within your dreams, there seems to be distance between the subject and the objects. However, when you wake up and remember your dream, you realize that the star you saw was no farther away than your eyelashes.

The truth is that the same applies to our daily experience. There is no distance between the Self as consciousness and the observed object. From our dual and relative perspective, we think that objective reality emerges in front of consciousness. However, what happens is that the reality of names and forms becomes present within consciousness. As we said, one of the sacred names of God in the Torah is *Ha Makom*, or "the Place." That is, God is the place or space where all experience occurs. Consciousness consists of an infinite space within which objects appear and disappear like bubbles in the ocean. If we previously thought we were distant witness of objects, it is enough to observe attentively to realize the intimacy of experience. Observation reveals the mysteries of reality.

Many are trapped in a dual conception of experience and think of infinite space as the subject and its content as the object. Such a belief does not allow us to transcend the relative duality of subject and object, manifested and unmanifested. To overcome this belief, we must discover that the objective reality and the infinite space where it manifests are made of the same raw material. The manifested is made of the same essential substance as the consciousness that perceives it. If we observe carefully, we will see that the only component of any object is perception, no matter if the object is physical, mental, or emotional. There is absolutely nothing within our experience that goes beyond perception and our knowledge of it.

Our respected scientific community investigates matter; however, no one knows what matter really is. The explanation offered by science resembles the information we have about Santa Claus. We know how he dresses and that he rides in a sleigh, he has a white beard, and he gives gifts to children at Christmas, but we do not know if he exists, and in fact, we doubt his existence.

Most human beings do not question the existence of solid matter. However, we have never known any object, animal, person, or star – we have only known our own perception of them. We know nothing but what we know, nor have we ever perceived anything except our perception. Every object that appears within the manifested reality shares exactly the same substance as the one who perceives it. Nevertheless, the conviction that there are two realities persists: one manifested and one unmanifested. We believe in a duality composed of two elements of radically different nature, subject and object. But in fact, experience is consciousness.

I hope I do not to disappoint anyone by saying that this is not a new discovery, as some satsangists try to present it. It is part of the very ancient *Advaita* revelation of Ādi Śaṅkarācārya in his famous *Brahma-jñānāvalī-mālā*:

ब्रह्म सत्यं जगन्मिथ्या जीवो ब्रह्मैव नापरः ।

brahma satyaṁ jagan mithyā
jīvo brahmaiva nāparaḥ

> Brahman is real. The universe is false. The *jīva* itself is Brahman: it is not different from Brahman.
>
> (*Brahma-jñānāvalī-mālā*, 20a)

Without ceasing to be what it is, even for a moment, consciousness assumes the form of a manifested diversity that we perceive as the universe. The Upanishadic *mahā-vākyas* such as "I am Brahman" (*ahaṁ brahmāsmi*) or "Thou art That" (*tat tvam asi*) show us that instead of being spectators of manifested reality, we are its very essence.

Enlightenment occurs when the boundaries between the manifested and the unmanifested collapse. It is the realization of being the Whole while, in reality, there is nothing. It means awakening to nothingness or beingness. The *Suñña Sutta*, part of the Pali Canon, relates that the monk Ānanda, Buddha's assistant, asked him:

> "The world is said to be empty, the world is empty, sir: In what sense is the world said to be empty?" The Buddha replied, "In so far as it is empty of an I or of anything pertaining to an I. Thus, it is said, Ānanda, that the world is empty."

Experience and consciousness are not two distinct elements, just as when we dream, the dreamer adopts the form of a dream world and creates a character to experience it. In our reality, it is perception that takes on the configuration of a universe. It is consciousness that assumes the form of a mind and a body. It is consciousness that becomes localized as a character in order to perceive the imagined world. Just as water takes the form of the glass or bottle that contains it, consciousness takes the form of thought in order to transform itself into a mind. Adopting the form of certain sensations, it manifests as a body. According to our mental interpretation, our body is a form; however, our body is first and foremost a series of sensations. The raw material of both the manifested and the unmanifested is one and the same. This substance is the essence of what we are.

Mantra 15

हिरण्मयेन पात्रेण सत्यस्यापिहितं मुखम् ।
तत्त्वं पूषन्नपावृणु सत्यधर्माय दृष्टये ॥

hiraṇmayena pātreṇa
satyasyāpihitaṁ mukham
tat tvaṁ pūṣann apāvṛṇu
satya-dharmāya dṛṣṭaye

The face of the Truth, in its dazzling splendor, is covered by a golden disc. O Sun! Please remove the disc and show yourself to this seeker of Truth.

Commentary:

This Upanishad has been preserved for generations by two lines of disciplic succession. The line begun by the sage Kāṇva preserved a version with 18 mantras. The last four of these are excluded by the Mādhyandina line, which maintains a version of only 14 mantras. In mantra 15, written by Dadhyannatharvana, the meter is *anuṣṭubh*, and the deity is the sun.

The important terms in this text are *pūṣan*, which means "one who nourishes." *Ṛṣi* means "seer" and refers to seers of the ultimate reality. *Mukham* means "the authentic nature of Truth." *Apihitam* means "it is covered." Hiraṇmayena refers to the golden hue and the term *pātreṇa* is for the circular form of the visible light that covers the Truth. Finally, the phrase *hiraṇmayena-pātreṇa* means "the golden refulgent light."

The *Bṛhad-āraṇyaka Upanishad* states:

तद्यत्तत्सत्यमसौ स आदित्यः—य एष एतस्मिन्मण्डले पुरुषः, यश्चायं दक्षिणेऽक्षन्पुरुषः; तावेतावन्योऽन्यस्मिन्प्रतिष्ठितौ; रश्मिभिरेषोऽस्मिन्प्रतिष्ठितः, प्राणैरयममुष्मिन्; स यदोत्क्रमिष्यन्भवति शुद्धमेवैतन्मण्डलं पश्यति; नैनमेते रश्मयः प्रत्यायन्ति ॥

tad yat tat satyam asau sa ādityaḥ—ya eṣa etasmin maṇḍale puruṣo yaś cāyaṁ dakṣiṇe 'kṣan puruṣas tāvetāv anyo 'nyasmin pratiṣṭhitau raśmibhir eṣo 'smin pratiṣṭhitaḥ prāṇair ayam amuṣmin sa yadotkramiṣyan bhavati

> *śuddham evaitan maṇḍalaṁ paśyati nainam ete raśmayaḥ pratyāyanti.*
>
> That which is *satya* is that sun, the being who is in that orb and the being who is in the right eye. These two rest on each other. The former rests on the latter through the rays, and the latter rests on the former through the function of the eyes. When someone is about to leave the body, the solar orb can be clearly seen. The rays no longer reach that person.
>
> (*Bṛhad-āraṇyaka Upanishad*, 5.5.2)

These last four mantras, 15–18, are prayers for seekers of Truth at the time of death. Each tradition has its own way of praying. Believers of different religions pray by imitating their respective prophets. Christians try to pray like Jesus and Muslims, like Muhammad. Jews pray three times a day like Abraham, Isaac, and Jacob. This means we have masses of parishioners imitating Buddha, Lao Tzu, Mahavira, Kabir, and so on. Many think they know how to pray, but perhaps they only pretend to pray. They may have learned the correct behavior during prayer, but their soul is not always in a state of prayer. While they pray with their body and lips, they do not pray with their soul. Our inner attitude of devotion and submission is the essential aspect. True prayer cannot be acquired with empty words and gestures. If it is not accompanied by an inner state of devotion, intention, gratitude, humility, and surrender, prayer is only a lifeless imitation of a ritual.

This mantra consists of prayers addressed to the Satyātman, or "Ātman of Truth," at the time of death. It does not necessarily refer to physical death, but the death of the ego. Vedantic prayer is an egoic effort to move from individual to transcendental consciousness. It is born from the dual dimension and aspires to merge into the Absolute. It is the part that aspires to harmonize with the Whole. It is the drop's desire to disappear into the ocean. It is the surrender of the personal to the universal.

Nowadays, "instructors" and "guides" of diverse self-help methodologies promote their methods, pointing out benefits and advantages. Many of them claim that their meditation techniques will fulfill their practitioners' most ambitious fantasies. However, the divine path is spiritual suicide, since it directly attacks the foundations of who we believe ourselves to be. It threatens the very basis of our egoic construction. The path to Truth will always be destructive because it aims to kill falsehood. The authentic path differs from the spiritual business that is sold at the fair of mundane mysticism. The former comes from enlightened beings who educate disciples, the latter from hucksters who serve customers who are always right.

The Sufi expression "to die before you die" may seem somewhat paradoxical. Rumi writes in his famous *Masnavi-ye-Ma'navi* (IV): "O, blessed are those who die before they die, for they have sniffed the perfume of this orchard's origin." In fact, this allegory refers to the extinction of our conditioned identity. It is a voluntary death, prior to physical death. This is what also Saul of Tarsus refers to in the Epistle to the Galatians (2:20): "And I no longer live, but Christ lives in me."

Thomas of Kempis, in his famous book, *Imitation of Christ* (2.12) alludes to this mystical death: "Be assured of this, that you must live a dying life. And the more completely you die to yourself, the more you begin to live for God."

We also read the following in Romans:

> For none of us lives for ourselves alone, and none of us dies for ourselves alone. If we live, we live for the Lord; and if we die, we die for the Lord. So, whether we live or die, we belong to the Lord.
>
> (New Testament, Romans 14:7–8)

> Now if we died with Christ, we believe that we will also live with him. For we know that since Christ was raised from the dead, he cannot die again; death no longer has mastery over him. The death he died, he died to sin once for all; but the life he lives, he lives to God.
>
> (New Testament, Romans 6:8–10)

Islam describes spiritual death with the word *fanā*, meaning "dissolution of the self" followed by the term *baqa*, or "subsistence in God." Such terminology comes from the Qur'an (*Sura* 55, *aleyas* 26–27): "All that is on earth will perish, only the Person of your Lord, full of majesty and splendor, will endure."

It is also based on a beautiful *hadith* by Muhammad, collected by Al Tirmidhi, which says: "Die before you die and ask for an account of yourself before you are asked for it."

The Persian poet and mystic Sanai wrote a *masnavi* poem in *The Enclosed Garden of the Truth* (*Hadiqat al haqiqa*).

> As long as you cling to your ego,
> you will wander right and left,
> day and night, for thousands of years;
> and when, after all that effort,
> you finally open your eyes,
> you will see your ego's inherent defects,
> wandering around itself like the ox on the mill;
> but, if, once freed from your ego,
> you finally get down to work,
> this door will open to you in two minutes.
> Bruise your ego for months and years on end;
> leave it for dead,
> and when you have finished it off, you will have reached eternal life.
> When you have killed your ego on the path,
> you will immediately be shown God's favor.

This mantra does not convey the prayers of an old man on his deathbed. Verses 15–18 are the final prayers of a very advanced seeker in deep meditation facing the last veil that covers ultimate reality. This person is an authentic *mumukṣutva* praying for the complete removal of the golden veil that covers the Truth.

Upanishadic literature does not contain repeated information or second-hand knowledge. It documents direct testimonies of those who transcended the personal and awakened to the Whole, of beings who died to what is temporary and were reborn in the eternal by transcending the relative dimension.

"O Sun! Please remove it."

We find a glimpse of this idea in the Rig Veda, when the sage Śrutavid Ātreya addresses the *devas* Mitrā and Varuṇa:

ऋतेन ऋतमपिहितं ध्रुवं वां सूर्यस्य यत्र विमुचन्त्यश्वान् ।
दश शता सह तस्थुस्तदेकं देवानां श्रेष्ठं वपुषामपश्यम् ॥

ṛtena ṛtam api hitaṁ dhruvaṁ
vāṁ sūryasya yatra vimucanty aśvān
daśa śatā saha tasthus tad ekaṁ
devānāṁ śreṣṭhaṁ vapuṣām apaśyam

The face of your divine Truth is permanently covered by Truth. It is there, where the gods unharness Sūrya's horses. There, ten thousand rays of light come together. There, I saw the *ekam tat* (a That), the most wonderful of all the *devas*.

(Rig Veda, 5.62.1)

There is a similar description in the *Chāndogya Upanishad*:

त इमे सत्याः कामा अनृतापिधानास्तेषाꣳ सत्यानाꣳ सतामनृतमपिधानं यो यो ह्यस्येतः प्रैति न तमिह दर्शनाय लभते ॥

ta ime satyāḥ kāmā anṛtāpidhānās teṣāṁ satyānāṁ satām anṛtamapidhānaṁ yo yo hy asy etaḥ praiti na tam iha darśanāya labhate.

But all these true desires are under a false cover. Though they rest on the Self, they are all false. This is why when relatives die, we do not see them again in this world.

(*Chāndogya Upanishad*, 8.3.1)

The seeker begs for the Truth to be shown to him. The *ṛṣi* knows that it is there, hidden behind a shining disk, unattainable for him.

Jesus' Father dwells in the heavens; He is not in the earthly, dual, and relative dimension, but beyond what is mental and mundane. Jesus addresses Him in the following way:

I praise you, Father, Lord of heaven and earth, because you have hidden these things from the wise and learned, and revealed them to little children.

(New Testament, Matthew, 11:25)

Truth remains hidden only to those who wish to perceive it through their mind. As Patañjali states:

द्रष्टा दृशिमात्रः शुद्धोऽपि प्रत्ययानुपश्यः ॥

draṣṭā dṛśimātraḥ śuddho 'pi pratyayānupaśyaḥ

> Those who see, though they are pure consciousness, see through the distortion of the mind.
>
> (*Yoga Sūtra*, 2.20)

Every observation made through lenses colored by our mental conditioning will necessarily be defective. Looking through a mind conditioned by political and religious organizations, cultures, and traditions, it is impossible to see what is true. If we use an instrument cluttered with concepts, conclusions, doctrines, conjectures, and prejudices, it is clearly impossible to access what really is. The mind is illusion and falsehood from its very roots, since it is based on a false conclusion about our very existence. The mind is the conviction that I am a disconnected entity, isolated from all things and all beings. Our efforts to reach Truth through falsehoods are futile.

Human beings do not perceive the world as it is, but as it seems to them. Many of us have the mistaken impression that we all live in the same world. However, the truth is that we all live and act in our own worlds. Instead of observing, we move through the world projecting our mental content and pasts onto what is observed. In Sanskrit, the mind is called *antaḥkaraṇa*, or "inner instrument," because through it, reality is perceived as something external. The mind consists of four different aspects: *manas*, *buddhi*, *citta*, and *ahaṅkāra*. *Manas* is the ability to think, *buddhi*, to discriminate, *citta*, to store impressions and memories, and *ahaṅkāra*, to preserve our own existence. *Ahaṅkāra*, the ego, takes credit for what has occurred and what is observed. In deeper dimensions, we find the subtle body, *sūkṣma-śarīra*, and in the more subconscious dimension, the causal body, *kāraṇa-śarīra*.

The deeper levels of consciousness are characterized by more subtle mental activity. The Vedic term *hiraṇyagarbha* refers to mental activity at all levels. To transcend the layers that cover *hiraṇyagarbha*, each one must be observed. In this meditative process, we stop at each level to observe each sheath. Only after becoming fully aware each sheath, do we continue to the next one. We progress from dense to subtle, from physical to causal. We gradually recognize both our conscious and unconscious egoism. Little by little, we cease to be victims of our own conditioning that we harbor in the depths of the mind.

"... show yourself to this seeker of Truth."

The last verses of the scripture respect the traditional Upanishadic style, which requires a certain coherence between beginning and end. Recall that the book began with: "All this, be it living beings or inert matter, is wrapped up by the Lord." Following this style, the work ends by addressing the Lord with this beautiful prayer.

To most readers, it may seem strange that the Vedic sage says that Truth is covered by a disk of golden light. It would seem more logical that the Truth is hidden behind darkness. However, one who has walked the entire path knows from personal experience that light not only illuminates but can also dazzle and, consequently, conceal. Light can both illuminate and blind. Under certain circumstances, it has the function of darkness. We cannot see the sun because it is too bright.

Looking at it objectively, the sun is not covered, but our eyes are too delicate to look at it. Because of our optical limitations, we conclude that the sun is covered by its brightness. Truth is not covered, but the instrument of observation alters what is observed. The mind is an instrument in which concepts, ideas, and conclusions are combined, laying the foundation for the illusory construct of the ego. The problem is that we see through a completely conditioned mind that only perceives what is apparent. We cannot adequately appreciate the present through an instrument that only sees memories and the past.

The more we are able to observe, and not just to think, the greater the clarity. The more the mind remains absent from our process of observation, the greater the luminosity. The splendor increases in direct proportion to the depths we are blessed with in meditation. At deeper levels of consciousness, our challenges will be very different. Darkness is a beginner's problem. For advanced seekers, it is light. In the beginning, the problem is twilight. In the end, it is blinding light. We take our first steps on the path on a dark, moonless night, but, as we move forward, the shining sun is closer to us than we are to ourselves.

The sun illuminates the interior of our homes without being inside them. Its light allows us to observe the walls, ornaments, furniture, and people in the rooms. In the same way, although the light of consciousness is not part of experience, it illuminates every experience. Every experience has this cognitive element that knows and is aware of the experience. Every experience becomes cognizable by the light of knowing. Nearly all human beings refer to the cognitive element of our experiences as "I." We know that we are the only knowers of our experiences. In investigating the "I," we discover that it is not "something" or "someone," but only the knowing of each experience. It is impossible to illuminate this conscious presence in the same way as objective experiences, because this presence is light. This cognitive element that knows each experience is only "knowing" or "being aware of." It is the very foundation of experience.

This knowing is the very essence of thoughts, feelings, sensations, and perceptions. Ultimately, this knowing is what we really are, our authentic nature. It is the space where every experience occurs, the knower of experiences and the very substance of each experience. It is possible to eliminate any object from our experience and it will continue to exist. We can eliminate everything and leave the experience completely without content. Then, we will say that there is absolutely nothing. But if it were possible to extract the cognitive element from the experience, it would be impossible to imagine what would remain.

If we could extract only the cognitive element of the experience, which is its very basis, there would be no experience. For to even say that absolutely nothing remains, the experience needs to be known. To say that we experience nothing, we also need to be aware of it. In fact, the light of consciousness, or knowing experience, is all it really is. The Hebrew revelation says *Ein od milbado*, or "there is nothing except Him." The light of consciousness can never know anything but itself. All that exists is infinite consciousness and all that is experienced is that same consciousness in different degrees and shades, just as H_2O at different temperatures is perceived as liquid, ice, snow, or steam. There has never been an object that exists outside of consciousness.

"The face of the Truth in its dazzling splendor is covered by a golden disc."

Many people remain at this stage for several reincarnations. This is a particularly difficult obstacle to overcome. Clearly, it is much easier to renounce suffering than happiness. Giving up our sinful tendencies is not as difficult as giving up holiness. Renouncing what is negative is easier than renouncing what is positive and good. Although both keep us equally imprisoned, the shiny platinum bars give us the illusory feeling that we possess something valuable. The beauty of the bars makes us forget that we that we are still imprisoned. On the path to Truth, it is not enough to renounce only what is negative. We also must transcend what is positive, which is generally more difficult to give up. When we become attached to something positive, it automatically becomes negative. This attachment is a barrier that limits our freedom and distances us from the Truth. Ultimately it is a matter of transcending both darkness and light. Truth resides beyond day and night. In the Jewish Passover Haggadah, there is a hymn written by Yanai, a sixth-century author from the land of Israel. The lyrics read:

קָרֵב יוֹם אֲשֶׁר הוּא לֹא יוֹם וְלֹא לַיְלָה
רָם הוֹדַע כִּי לְךָ הַיּוֹם אַף לְךָ הַלַּיְלָה
שׁוֹמְרִים הַפְקֵד לְעִירְךָ כָּל הַיּוֹם וְכָל הַלַּיְלָה
תָּאִיר כְּאוֹר יוֹם חֶשְׁכַת לַיְלָה.

Soon will come a day that is neither day nor night,
Elevated One, make it known that Yours is the day and Yours is also the night,
Appoint guards to Your city all day and all night,
Illuminate the darkness of the night like the light of the day.

Overcoming darkness and light, we awaken to the absolute plane or the reality of the One without a second.

न तद्भासयते सूर्यो न शशाङ्को न पावकः ।
यद्गत्वा न निवर्तन्ते तद्धाम परमं मम ॥

na tad bhāsayate sūryo
na śaśāṅko na pāvakaḥ
yad gatvā na nivartante
tad dhāma paramaṁ mama

That which the sun does not illuminate, nor the moon, nor fire, that is my supreme abode. Having attained that, there is no return.

(Bhagavad Gita, 15.6)

Then, there is an awakening to the dimension of the Absolute, which has no duality or relativity. It does not allow divisions such as darkness and light, death and life, prosaic and sacred, suffering and happiness, and so on. Awakening to non-dual reality means dissolving conflict. Masters from diverse traditions have referred to the non-dual in many ways. In the Bible, Zechariah states:

וְהָיָה בַּיּוֹם הַהוּא לֹא יִהְיֶה אוֹר יְקָרוֹת וְקִפָּאוֹן. וְהָיָה יוֹם אֶחָד
הוּא יִוָּדַע לַה' לֹא יוֹם וְלֹא לָיְלָה וְהָיָה לְעֵת עֶרֶב יִהְיֶה אוֹר.
(זכריה י"ד, ו'-ז')

On that day, there shall be neither sunlight nor moonlight, but there shall be a continuous day only the Lord knows when—of neither day nor night, and there shall be light in the evening.

(Zechariah, 14:6–7)

The human mind resists transcending goodness. It is only when we try to take a few steps that we become aware of our chains. Human beings will not be truly free until they sincerely desire and decide to be free. When it comes to freedom, there are no good chains. At this point on the path, a great conflict between our lower nature and our divine nature arises. The temptation to adorn the prison cell and our craving for freedom are pitted against each other. In general, it is more difficult to renounce gold chains than iron ones. This conflict gives birth to the prayer in this verse.

Within a dual reality, we will only find relative happiness and freedom. We experience the freedom of a weekend or a vacation, but the absolute and most important freedom is being what we really are. The path from 'here to here' that leads to the Self is riddled with luminous temptations. The road back to the place we never left is overflowing with fireworks and momentary distractions.

The grosser a pleasure, the easier it is to abandon. Subtle appetites are more difficult to overcome. The most difficult are the mystical pleasures that originate in our astral intimacy. Pleasures that come from more subtle planes convince us that we have reached the goal, that our long pilgrimage is over. To leave such "achievements" behind, our willpower is of little use. For there is no willpower capable of transcending them. Colorful and provisional mystical experiences can stagnate us, awake our vanity, and persuade us that we are great enlightened beings. The energy to continue on the path from this point onwards can only come from surrender. After having done everything humanly possible, only divine grace can help. The sage invokes it in this mantra.

Willpower and determination are very useful to transcend darkness, but not light. Transcending darkness involves sacrifices; however, human effort is insufficient to overcome the light. Through much striving, the sage has succeeded in leaving darkness behind and reaching the light. This is as far as our efforts can take us. Meditation leads us from darkness to light, but it is not enough to transcend the light.

ॐ असतोमा सद्गमय ।
तमसोमा ज्योतिर्गमय ।
मृत्योर्मामृतं गमय ॥
ॐ शान्ति शान्ति शान्तिः ॥

oṁ asato mā sad gamaya
tamaso mā jyotir gamaya
mṛtyor mā amṛtaṁ gamaya
oṁ śānti śānti śāntiḥ

Lead me from inexistence to existence. Lead me from darkness to light. Lead me from death to immortality. *Oṁ* Peace Peace Peace.

(*Pavamāna Mantra* from *Bṛhad-āraṇyaka Upanishad*, 1.3.28)

From this point on, we depend on divine grace. All that remains is to pray and completely surrender ourselves to existence. You have reached this stage through study, techniques, methods, practice, determination, and willpower. But here you will be obliged to pray with full and absolute surrender. That is why, at the end of the Upanishad, after having understood what a human being can do to harmonize with the Whole, you can only implore grace and surrender yourself into the hands of God.

> To what shore would you cross, O my heart?
> there is no traveler before you, there is no road:
> ...
> There is no water; no boat, no boatman.
> There is not even a rope to tow the boat, nor someone to pull it.
> ...
> Be strong, and enter into your own body:
> for there, your foothold is firm.
>
> There,
> there is no rain,
> no ocean, no sun, no shadow.
>
> There,
> there is neither creation nor destruction,
> neither living nor dying,
> nor the trace of sadness or joy.

There,
there is neither solitude nor meditation.
Nothing is measured, nothing is wasted,
nothing is lightweight, nothing is heavy.

There, no one is powerful or weak.
There, there is neither night nor day.
There, there is no water, no air, no fire.
There, only the true guru
permeates everything.

Kabir

MANTRA 16

पूषन्नेकर्षे यम सूर्य प्राजापत्य व्यूह रश्मीन् समूह तेजः ।
यत्ते रूपं कल्याणतमं तत्ते पश्यामि योऽसावसौ पुरुषः सोऽहमस्मि ॥

pūṣann ekarṣe yama sūrya prājāpatya
vyūha raśmīn samūha
tejo yat te rūpaṁ kalyāṇa-tamaṁ
tat te paśyāmi yo 'sāvasau puruṣaḥ so 'ham asmi

O nutrient! O only seer! O commander of Truth! O enlightening sun! O son of Prajāpati! Withdraw your rays and collect your bright light, so that I may behold your most glorious form. The Puruṣa within you is me.

Commentary:

"O enlightening sun!"

This verse was revealed by the *ṛṣi* Dadhyannathurvaṇa and it was written in the Vedic meter *uṣṇih*. The sage's prayer addresses the solitary traveler of the sky, also known as the controller and nourisher of vital energy (*prāṇa*) and essence (*rasa*) of everything, the son of the creator Prajāpati.

In Greek mythology, the personification of the sun was Helios, one of the titan gods and son of Hyperion and Theia. His siblings were Selene (the moon) and Eos (the dawn). In the Inca empire, the sun was the main deity on the celestial plane, called Inti, a term borrowed from the Puquina language. In India, the Vedas proclaimed that the sun god is the spiritual master of the sage Yājñavalkya, the compiler of the *Śukla Yajur Veda Saṁhitā*, which includes the *Īśāvāsya Upanishad.*

At first glance, this prayer is addressed to Sūrya, the solar deity, using one of his many sacred names, Pūṣan. This name appears in the *Yajur Veda* and is derived from the verb *puṣ*, meaning "to make prosper." The Vedic sages considered Pūṣan to be the sustainer and nourisher of the cosmic manifestation. He is the source of luminous energy in the cosmos.

The Vedas refer to Pūṣan's revelatory power as "sight or vision." In the Rig Veda, we find eight hymns dedicated to him that invoke him to protect cattle. In the *Taittirīya Saṁhitā*, consisting of eight *kāṇḍas*, we find a narrative of Rudra being excluded from a sacrificial ceremony. Furious, he shot an arrow that pierced the offering and broke Pūṣan's teeth just as he was about to eat an oblation. This story gave Lord Śiva one of his names, Pūṣa-danta-hara, "the one who took out Pūṣan's teeth." Another name is Pūṣa-asuhṛd, or "the one not much liked by Pūṣan." This story is also in the *Rāmāyaṇa* and *Mahābhārata*, as well as other *Puranas*.

Pūṣan is one of the twelve *ādityas*, or forms of Sūrya, the sun god. Lord Brahmā mentioned the 108 names of the sun god to the sages. The *Śrīmad-bhāgavatam* (12.11.27–49) lists his sacred names and they are also mentioned in the *Mahābhārata* ("*Vana parva*," section 3.10).

According to modern science, the sun is a star at the center of the solar system. It is a large hot ball of gas that shines due to electromagnetic radiation. Our planetary system is solar because eight planets, including the Earth, orbit the sun. The sun is the only body in the solar system that emits its own light, which comes from the thermonuclear fusion of hydrogen and its transformation into helium. After the sun exhausts all its hydrogen, it will not send any light to our planet, and Earth will become an inert rock.

Clearly, the sage is not praying to what we think of as the sun, the Greek god Helios, or the Inca god Inti. He is addressing the sun as the center of our existence. Each of us is a center around which thoughts, ideas, conclusions, memories, emotions, feelings, sensations, and perceptions revolve. The center of consciousness is like the sun and our activities are like the orbits of the planets. According to Newton's theory, the planets move thanks to the attraction of the Sun's gravitational force. Their motion is real, but it depends on the sun. It is not independent, since it borrows its beingness from the center.

Undoubtedly, objective reality is real and it exists. Objects and bodies exist, but they do not exist independently. Objective reality borrows its existence from consciousness, which is the *El Chai ve'Kayam*, which in Hebrew means "God as life and existence itself." The Rambam (Rabbi Moshe Ben Maimon) addressed this topic in his famous *Mishneh Torah*:

> יְסוֹד הַיְּסוֹדוֹת וְעַמּוּד הַחָכְמוֹת, לֵידַע שֶׁיֵּשׁ שָׁם מָצוּי רִאשׁוֹן. וְהוּא מַמְצִיא כָּל הַנִּמְצָא; וְכָל הַנִּמְצָאִים מִן שָׁמַיִם וָאָרֶץ וּמַה שֶּׁבֵּינֵיהֶם, לֹא נִמְצְאוּ אֵלָּא מֵאֲמִתַּת הִמָּצְאוֹ. וְאִם יַעֲלֶה עַל הַדַּעַת שֶׁהוּא אֵינוּ מָצוּי, אֵין דָּבָר אַחֵר יָכוֹל לְהִמָּצְאוֹת.
>
> (משנה תורה, הלכות יסודי התורה, פרק א', הלכות א'-ב')

> The foundation of all foundations and the pillar of wisdom is to know that there is a primary existence who brought into being all existence. All that exists, from the heavens, the earth, and what is between them came into existence only from the truth of His existence. If one would imagine that He does not exist, no other thing could possibly exist.
>
> (*Mishneh Torah, Hilchot Yesodei Ha'torah*, "Foundations of the Torah," 1.1–2)

This is also mentioned in *Pirkei Avot,* or "Ethics of the Fathers":

> רַבִּי אֶלְעָזָר אִישׁ בַּרְתּוֹתָא אוֹמֵר: תֶּן לוֹ מִשֶּׁלּוֹ, שֶׁאַתָּה וְשֶׁלְּךָ שֶׁלּוֹ. וְכֵן בְּדָוִד הוּא אוֹמֵר (דברי הימים א' כ"ט, י"ד): כִּי מִמְּךָ הַכֹּל, וּמִיָּדְךָ נָתַנּוּ לָךְ.
>
> (פרקי אבות ג', ז')
>
> "Rabbi Elazar of Bartotha said: 'Give Him of what is His, for you and that which is yours are His'; and in this way David says (I Chronicles, 29:14): 'For everything comes from You, and from Your own hand have we given you.'"
>
> (*Pirkei Avot*, 3.7)

We are a presumed peripheral activity around an omnipresent center. The appreciation of the sun in ancient cultures reflects the yearning of human beings to return to their original center. Just as the solar center is the source of energy and the driver of other renewable energies, our activity, whether energetic, emotional, mental, or physical, borrows its existence from the center. This verse metaphorically refers to *ātman* as the sun, the nourisher, seer, controller, the one center of all things and all beings.

The retroprogressive process is a search for the center and an attempt to center ourselves. Most humans are eccentric because they live off-centered. Instead of orbiting around our inner sun, we revolve around fantasies, dreams, illusions, wishes, desires, and ambitions. Although we believe that the center, which we call ego, resides within us, we are unable to find it. No one has ever found their ego. Our inexplicable apathy allows us to live without seeking who we are, which reinforces our belief that a private center exists.

We are pure consciousness free of objective attributes. But because we have been locked in our mental cage for so long, we have forgotten how to fly. Confused about who we are, we have assumed false identities as separate and independent entities. We identify with the egoic phenomenon of a "thought-I" even though it is very different to *think* "I" than to *be* "I."

"O only seer!"

This mantra refers to the ultimate Truth as *ekarṣi*, a term meaning "the only seer." To understand its meaning, let us clarify that all experience has a cognitive element, which is the knowing of the experience. The cognitive element, or knowingness, is the light of consciousness. Although it is the knowing of every experience, it is not an integral part of the experience itself since it cannot be located as another object within the experience. We usually baptize this cognitive element as "I." All human beings know themselves to be the only knower of their most intimate experiences. But when we investigate this cognitive element, we discover that it is not "something" endowed with qualities. It is completely devoid of attributes and objective dimensions. Such a cognitive element is only "knowing" or "cognizing"; it is the light of consciousness, the basis and foundation of all experience.

Consciousness, or our authentic nature, is the space where all experience occurs. It is the very substance of experience and through which experience is known. It is the only immutable element that, if we try to extract it from experience, experience would have no foundation. Objects can be eliminated without experience as such being affected. If we tear our every object from experience and leave it empty, we could say that there is nothing that lacks content. But this would still be an experience, because it would not have been destroyed. It is impossible to destroy the screen from inside the film. If it were possible to eliminate the cognitive element of the experience, we could not even imagine what would remain afterwards. If we extracted only the knowing from an experience, there would simply be no experience because knowingness is its foundation. Without the presence of the cognitive element, we cannot realize that there is no content.

God is the only knower, because the cognitive element can never know anything separate from itself. It knows only knowing, cognizes only cognizing, and perceives only perceiving. All that exists is infinite consciousness. All experiences, mental or physical, are different shades of the same consciousness. It is impossible for there to be an object independent of consciousness. God is *ekarṣi*, the only seer and experiencer of all experience.

"O commander of Truth!"

Obsessed with finding our ego, we look for it within ourselves. However, our true nature cannot be found in objective reality. To the mind, consciousness devoid of attributes is simply emptiness. This feeling of emptiness comes from a fruitless search for the ego.

However, the mind is very sophisticated and when it perceives such emptiness, it claims any peace or silence as its own. The separate "I" reappears by objectifying emptiness as one of its most precious achievements and possessions. When the ego thinks about emptiness, it incorporates it into its objective reality as a mental and emotional object. It conceptualizes this emptiness and transforms it into a "mental nothingness." This is one of the mind's main strategies for creating mental meditation, mental enlightenment, and for transforming God into a mental and sentimental object.

Mental reality is not real; it is subjective. Absolute reality cannot be achieved through subjective reality. Any reaction to the void will be irrefutable proof that emptiness has vanished and that the separate "thought-I" has returned, this time with its own version of emptiness. The egoic response means that emptiness is like an objective stimulus. Along with the reappearance of the ego, illusionary emptiness will simply vanish. The authenticity of an achieved nothingness is very doubtful, because it is only a conceptualization or verbalization of emptiness.

Authentic emptiness can be conceived of but not

perceived by the egoic phenomenon. If we can think about emptiness, appreciate it, and admire it, then it is not real emptiness; it is objectified emptiness. Instead of identifying with an independent entity–subject, we should allow attention to return by itself to its source and origin. Then we will find emptiness itself and there will not be a separate "I" that perceives it.

Nothingness will be revealed only after the ego fails in a long search. The ego begins to evaporate when it becomes disenchanted for not finding what it sought. Imagine that your living room has had a gray carpet for many years. Your partner wants to surprise you and replaces it with a brown one. The next time you enter your apartment, you will not see the brown carpet; you will see the absence of the gray carpet. You will see what is missing instead of what is there. Similarly, the early stages of emptiness are the lack of ego. Although the ego has disappeared, it has not yet been fully transcended because you are attached to its absence. It is an emptiness that is the opposite of objective reality or its negative aspect; it is the absence of an objective universe.

The search begins in the acceptance of a false and illusory center. It will pass through the disappearance of that center, then the realization of being all, and finally centralization. In the first stage, we believe we are something, then we experience ourselves as the essence of everything. Finally, objects are revealed to be non-existent; therefore, there are no things to be the essence of. It is an identificatory process from what we think we are to what we really are; from thinking "I" to being "I."

The emptiness that Buddha describes, or *śūnyatā*, is more than the absence of ego. Discovering our core is not finding something. It is finding ourselves. It is not reaching our center but centering ourselves. As we center ourselves, pairs of opposites disappear.

Existence fully unfolds only when the non-existence of matter is revealed. In centralization, we disappear as a particular nucleus to be reborn as the center of life itself. Personality is based on a false center, while individuality is the expression of genuine centering. Then, we cease to act from our private center and our activities become transcendental.

Along with centralization, both the personality and the witness will dissolve into the infinite ocean of nothingness. Our actions will be charged with extraordinary power as all of existence is behind them. Just as every object borrows its reality and existence from the sun or consciousness at the center, our actions will be backed by existence itself. Not only our words, but even our presence and silences will emanate from the sun of suns.

The central core, or sun of life, will only reveal itself when we lose ourselves in the void without reacting. To do so requires courage because we must watch ourselves agonize and die, in front of our own eyes, and do nothing about it.

וַיֹּאמֶר לֹא תוּכַל לִרְאֹת אֶת פָּנָי כִּי לֹא יִרְאַנִי הָאָדָם וָחָי.
(שמות ל"ג, כ')

> And he said: "But you cannot see My face, for a man shall not see Me and live."
>
> (Exodus, 33:20)

"Withdraw your rays..."

As explained in the previous mantra, after leaving behind darkness, it is essential to transcend light. To access the Absolute, we must overcome relative duality. As long as we move within the apparent subject–object reality, we will live as subjects in conflict with objects.

On the dual plane, we perceive ourselves as beings that are fractured, divided, incomplete, and limited. This misperception induces a deep dissatisfaction and encourages us to try to complete ourselves by acquiring objects. We strive in vain to eliminate our deep discontent by trying to possess people and goods in hopes of finding fulfillment through them.

Living our lives as individualized subjects, we constantly avoid what is undesirable and pursue what is desirable. We avoid the discomfort of darkness and pursue the comfort of light. We want to enlarge the bright side of the moon and shrink the dark side. But this is impossible because as one side expands, so does the other. As the darkness shrinks, so does the light: both are inseparable aspects of the same moon.

We try to avoid suffering and strive for happiness. We flee from the negative and seek the positive. This attitude of attraction and rejection toward pairs of opposites brings misery and suffering. Our endeavors fail due to the transitory nature of both the object and the subject, an impermanence that Buddhism calls *anicca* or *anitya*. Both the seeker and what is sought change constantly, which makes it difficult to obtain and maintain what is desired. This constant mutation causes changes in subject–object relationships and makes it impossible to find bliss.

Dual reality is merely a belief that originates out of ignorance. From an absolute perspective, subject and object are two aspects of the same consciousness. Enlightenment means recognizing the common nature of both, as different rays of the same sun. When we suppose that they are separate phenomena, subject and object seem to distance themselves and this gives birth to the illusory experience of an objective reality of multiplicity. It triggers the cognitive process that defines knower, known, and knowledge. The definition of the observer also includes the observed object, as well as the observation and space where all this takes place.

> That which is in itself must become an object, to mankind, must arrive at consciousness, thus becoming for man. What has become an object to him is the same as what he is in himself through the becoming objective of this implicit being, man first becomes for himself; he is made double, is retained and not changed into another.

> For example, man is thinking, and thus he thinks out thoughts. In this way it is in thought alone that thought is object; reason produces what is rational: reason is its own object.
>
> (*Lectures on the Philosophy of History* by G.W. Hegel – Introduction)

"...collect your bright light..."

In his prayer addressed to the "nourisher," whose rays maintain the dual cosmic manifestation, the sage requests: "collect your bright light." In other words, gather up all of this dual manifestation that is nourished by your light. Gather both pain and pleasure, distress and happiness, evil and goodness, defeat and triumph, darkness and light. Collect the rays that nourish and maintain the illusory dual dimension with both object and subject, that is, collect even the subject, or the "I," that is part of relative reality. Seekers aim at the direct realization of the source and origin of everything. They long for access to the direct perception of that which is prior to all that is. They aspire to what only those who are willing to pay the price of their own "I" have access to.

At the end of the path, you realize that losing yourself is the best way to find yourself. Losing yourself as what you think you are, in order to find yourself as what you really are. Loosing yourself as a "thought-I," in order to find yourself again as beingness.

To a certain extent, we are talking about dying in the dual to be reborn in the Absolute. From the Middle East, more than two thousand years ago, we hear the echo of these blessed words of Jesus in the New Testament:

> Then Jesus said to his disciples, "Whoever wants to be my disciple must deny themselves and take up their cross and follow me. For whoever wants to save their life will lose it, but whoever loses their life for me will find it."
>
> (New Testament, Matthew, 16:24–25)

These words touched the heart of Saul of Tarsus, who would later be called Paul. Only after long years of surrender to his master and walking the path of the spirit, he wrote this reply, from prison in Rome:

> I have been crucified with Christ and I no longer live, but Christ lives in me. The life I now live in the body, I live by faith in the Son of God, who loved me and gave himself for me.
>
> (Galatians, 2:20)

Paul's reply to his master is phrase for phrase:

Jesus: "Take up their cross."
Paul: "I have been crucified with Christ."

Jesus: "Deny themselves."

Paul: "I no longer live, but Christ lives in me."

Jesus: "Follow me."
Paul: "The life I now live in the body, I live by faith in the Son of God."

When Paul says, "I have been crucified with Christ and I no longer live, but Christ lives in me," it is understood that the subject, or the "I," that no longer lives in him is the ego, which has been crucified with its master. Paul says:

> For we know that our old self was crucified with him so that the body ruled by sin might be done away with, that we should no longer be slaves to sin.
> (Romans, 6:6)

After his encounter with Jesus and his teachings, Paul negates himself, renouncing his separate "I." This negation, together with the overcoming of the object, are indispensable requisites for accessing Reality. In order for this to happen, we have to realize that we ourselves are an integral part of the relative world we are trying to transcend. We are not separate entities from the dual and illusory dimension we wish to overcome. We are part of it. It is utterly impossible for dual reality to be transcended and Truth to be realized as long as the "I" persists, even as a supposedly enlightened entity.

"The Puruṣa within you is me."

Throughout history, many have misinterpreted the teachings of great non-dualistic masters. They have made the mistake of thinking that Vedantic teachings say that objects do not exist. The great Upanishadic sages of antiquity did not deny the existence of objects, but maintained that objects cannot exist independently from consciousness. This should not be confused with Plato's *orthotex*, or "the correction of representation." That is to say, even though objects cannot exist independently, it does not mean that formless matter only acquires form on the eidetic plane. Things lack independent existence and are perceived as separate only because of relationships with them. Relationships lead to diversity, which is an immediate consequence of thought.

Relationships, duality, thought, and language are reflections of the mind, therefore, objects and things are synonymous with thoughts and ideas. A thought is a differentiated appreciation of information that vibrates in the infinite ocean of consciousness. Such information is detected, stored, and appropriated by the sense of "I." This means that every relationship consists of both verbal and mental activity. The existence of the egoic phenomenon depends entirely on its relationship with otherness, that is, people, objects, and ideas. The ego emanates from otherness; it emerges from others. Relationships are mirrors that reflect us.

The history of our life is the history of our relationships.

Relationships are mirrors in which we can observe ourselves and discover ourselves. It is only possible to relate to objects that are separate from us. To perceive them as separate, it is necessary to think about them. Trees, chairs, pencils, and people appear to exist objectively, but only when the thought of that object appears. Observing empirical reality, free of thought, allows us to access a reality of sensations and perceptions.

When we walk through the forest, we recognize trees of different colors, sizes, and textures. Only when we conceptualize and verbalize the word *tree* is it possible to recognize a tree as an object that is separate from other things. In reality, all conceptualizations and verbalizations emanate from and merge into consciousness. They do not give information from an external dual universe but create it. If we look around without the intervention of thought, the idea "tree" will not appear.

We perceive objects as independent because of their relationships to other objects. I conceive of a tree because there is an infinity of objects that are not trees. I perceive the objective universe as "not-me" because there is someone I call "me." We must just observe our reflection in the mirror of the relationship, rather than manipulating the experience that appears in the mirror. Manipulation is futile and unnecessary because appearances do not have an existence independent from consciousness. They are mere appearances in consciousness.

The matter of independent objects is just a result of thought manifesting and disappearing in consciousness.

Therefore, only the revealing observation is necessary. Observation allows us to discover that all conflictive relationships are a consequence of focusing on our mental activity rather than on our true nature, which is the space in where all relationships take place. Observation reveals that our opinions, ideas, and concepts about others are more related to our definition of "I" than to others. Both the definition of the subject, or "I," and of the object, or "the other," emerge simultaneously as two sides of the same coin. The perceptions of selfhood and otherness emerge together. They are interdependent. For example, to perceive a bottle as an independent object, we must conceptualize both the bottle and everything that is not a bottle at the same time.

The independent or isolated "I" can only be perceived in comparison with the "non-I." Sameness can only exist when contrasted with otherness. Conflicts depend on the blind belief that objects have an independent existence. Thought creates illusory separation. Language often bases its definitions on what something is not. Conceptualizations are defined by their opposite. Light is light because it is not darkness. Good is good because it is not bad. If there is a here, it is because there is a there. Beauty exists because ugliness is absent, just as intelligence exists because stupidity is absent. Even much spiritual terminology comes from an emphasis on conceptualizing and thus belongs on the dualistic platform. For example, something spiritual is not material, something holy is not demonic, sin is not virtue. Other examples are self as the opposite of non-self, duality versus non-duality, and consciousness as the opposite of objective diversity.

> כַּאֲשֶׁר הַדָּבָר הַטּוֹב נוֹדָע מֵהֶפְכּוֹ יְדִיעָה אֲמִתִּית, וְכֵן כָּל הַדְּבָרִים נִקְנֶה הַיְּדִיעָה בָּהֶם מִן הַהֵפֶךְ, כִּי מִן מַרְאֶה הַשָּׁחוֹר יָכוֹל לָדַעַת מַרְאֶה הַלָּבָן שֶׁהוּא הֶפְכּוֹ, וְכֵן כָּל הַהֲפָכִים, מִן הָאֶחָד נִקְנֶה הַיְּדִיעָה בַּהֶפֶךְ שֶׁלּוֹ. וּמֻסְכָּם הוּא כִּי 'יְדִיעַת הַהֲפָכִים הוּא אֶחָד'. וּבִשְׁבִיל זֶה אָמְרוּ בְּעַרְבֵי פְּסָחִים (פסחים קט"ז, א') בַּהַגָּדָה: 'מַתְחִיל בִּגְנוּת וּמְסַיֵּם בְּשֶׁבַח'. וְלָמָּה מַתְחִיל בִּגְנוּת, רַק שֶׁמִּפְּנֵי שֶׁאֵין לַשֶּׁבַח הַכָּרָה אֲמִתִּית רַק מִן הַהֵפֶךְ. וְלָכֵן אֵין לְפָרֵשׁ עִנְיַן הַגְּאֻלָּה הָאַחֲרוֹנָה, אִם לֹא שֶׁנְּבָאֵר עִנְיַן הַגָּלוּת וְהַחֻרְבָּן, שֶׁבָּזֶה יִוָּדַע הַטּוֹב וְהַתְּשׁוּעָה שֶׁאָנוּ מְקַוִּין.
>
> (מהר"ל, נצח ישראל, א')

Just as a real knowledge of the good can be acquired from knowing its opposite, and all things are known from their opposite, like how seeing black, one can know what white looks like, so it is with all the opposites, from one, the knowledge of its opposite is acquired. And it is accepted that "the knowledge of the opposites is one." And for this reason, this is said in the chapter "The nights of Passover" (*Psachim*, 116) about the Haggadah: 'it starts with defamation and ends with praise' and why does it start with defamation? Just because praise does not gain true recognition without its opposite. Therefore, the matter of the last redemption is not to be explained, unless we explain the matter of the exile and destruction, in which the good and salvation we hope for will be clarified.

(Maharal, *Netzach Yisrael*, 1)

A concept is meaningless without its opposite. Without the concept of death, we would not understand the concept of life. We can also mention the immanence of thought, since every concept contains its opposite. The concept of life is within the concept of death. Finally, verbalized concepts acquire their meaning through relationships. The concept of being is found in its relationship to non-being. Without thought, duality would not exist; therefore, duality cannot be considered real.

नासतो विद्यते भावो नाभावो विद्यते सतः ।
उभयोरपि दृष्टोऽन्तस्त्वनयोस्तत्त्वदर्शिभिः ॥

nāsato vidyate bhāvo
nābhāvo vidyate sataḥ
ubhayor api dṛṣṭo 'ntas
tv anayos tattva-darśibhiḥ

The knowers of Truth have concluded that what is non-existent has no permanence, and what exists does not cease to be. These seers have concluded it by studying the nature of both.

(Bhagavad Gita, 2.16)

The dual platform is created by conceptualizing and verbalizing a sense of "I." Many development methods include "spiritual" practices that assume that the dual platform is real. They offer techniques for proper interaction between "me" and "others." They teach all kinds of meditations for a deluded "I" that aspires to be an enlightened "I," or for an ignorant "I" that aspires to be an awakened "I." These methods only treat the symptoms and ignore the disease. A method based on a false premise cannot be correct. It is essential is to realize that "I" and "others" are mere appearances in order to recognize that consciousness is our true nature.

As egoic phenomena, we are only thoughts and ideas. Therefore, we never meet, nor do we love each other, nor do we fight. Identification with a thought creates separation, disconnection, and independence. The human ego is a mental construct, but we are not the thoughts. We are the consciousness or space where thoughts appear and disappear, come and go.

All humans are mental stories that are foundations for a separate "I." We tell ourselves a story about who we, and this includes others. I am a spiritual being because others are materialistic; I am sad because others are happy; I am smart because others are stupid; I am on a path that leads to God because others are not. I am as I am because I am not as I should be or as I am expected to be. The idea I have of others depends entirely on what I believe about myself. The story we tell and believe about ourselves and others is based on a relationship of opposites, that is, conflict. To be smart, idiots are necessary; to be beautiful, there must be some ugly people; to be good a person, I need evil people. If the opposite is missing, neither identity nor separation is possible.

Any narrative about ourselves is illusory because it is only mental activity and not absolute reality. There are no objects or people with an independent existence outside of thought. The idea of the independent "I" creates individual entities. Such ego-centered thinking contains both the "I" and the "other." Internally, it separates what I am from what I could or should be. Externally, it divides the "I" and the "other." Objective separation requires an otherness that defines the opposite of what we think we are. Fracture and conflict will perpetuate as long as we define who we are through thought instead of recognizing consciousness as our reality.

Consciousness is prior to the mind. However, in trying to conceptualize or verbalize it, we are entering into a relationship on the relative platform. It is impossible to relate to consciousness as an object because it lacks attributes and, thus, cannot be framed within any kind of relationship. Dualism is illusory in the sense that it is not part of an empirical reality; its existence is mental. When realizing naked consciousness, objective reality ceases to be perceived as verbalized concepts. What is conscious of every experience is not thought but consciousness. Thoughts, ideas, emotions, and feelings do not listen, speak, or act. Consciousness is the observation of experiences, their source, and their origin, the space where they occur, and their substance.

> שְׂאוּ מָרוֹם עֵינֵיכֶם וּרְאוּ מִי בָרָא אֵלֶּה הַמּוֹצִיא בְמִסְפָּר צְבָאָם
> לְכֻלָּם בְּשֵׁם יִקְרָא מֵרֹב אוֹנִים וְאַמִּיץ כֹּחַ אִישׁ לֹא נֶעְדָּר.
> (ישעיהו מ', כ"ו)

> Lift high your eyes and see: Who created these? He who brings out their host by count, who calls them each by name: by His great might and vast power, not one fails to appear.
>
> (Isaiah, 40:26)

The thought or idea "you" simultaneously creates the object and the subject. I marginalize the other, separating and defining myself as "I." Through conceptualizations, I demarcate mental boundaries that I consider real. To confirm these boundaries, I compare myself to an antagonistic otherness and maintain a conflict with it. To be beautiful, there must be others who are ugly. To be able to consider myself sincere, there must necessarily be hypocrites.

Conflictive interactions cause us distress. But if instead of paying attention to what happens on the objective platform, we focus on our present experience, we will realize that this antagonistic "other" lives in our mind–body complex as thoughts, emotions, and sensations. Our knowledge of the "other" can only occur through the mind.

Conflict with an antagonistic object comes from identifying with thought. If we observe, we will see that mental and emotional activity has no relationship to what we really are. If we cease to identify with the thinking subject, the conflict with the object disappears.

If we let go of thoughts and emotions, we remain as conscious unconceptualized space. In such a space, relationships and conflicts dissolve. It is in the recognition of consciousness that both thoughts and emotions are revealed as integral parts of consciousness itself. Mental and emotional activity does not happen to someone, they simply happen in that conscious space.

Likewise, conscious space and mental activity are made of the same substance. Both thoughts and feelings are consciousness. By recognizing consciousness, the boundaries between the activity manifesting within the space and the space itself disappear. Then, the "I" and the "other" merge and the conflict between them vanishes.

Mental and emotional activities are temporary appearances in consciousness; consciousness is what we really are. Recognizing it exposes the falsehood of duality and conflict.

Obviously, thought cannot transcend thought. The mind cannot go beyond the mind. So instead of striving, let us choose to recognize consciousness as what we really are.

Thought is how consciousness knows itself. So there is no need to change appearances, but to just observe.

Instead of manipulating what is apparent, just observe what is. Observing reveals to us that all objects and beings are thoughts or ideas.

There is no need to manipulate the thoughts or feelings that are reflected in the mirror of relationships because these are an integral part of consciousness. Methods or techniques will not help us reach pure consciousness, because it is already our eternal nature.

We can compare consciousness, or that knowing element of each experience, with a mirror. Consciousness witnesses all experience, reflecting what is in front of it. Everything reflected occurs in front of the mirror and not in it. Wisdom consists in being a mirror, or completely "disidentifying" from everything that is reflected. Experiences appear and disappear, come and go, but the mirror remains unchanged. The mirror does not retain past reflections but only shows what happens now. Enlightened ones live like a mirror, without yesterday or tomorrow. They are filled with the present experience, and when it disappears, no residue remains.

MANTRA 17

वायुरनिलममृतमथेदं भस्मांतꣳ शरीरम् ।
ॐ क्रतो स्मर कृतꣳ स्मर क्रतो स्मर कृतꣳ स्मर ॥

vāyur anilam amṛtam
athedaṁ bhasmāntaṁ śarīram
oṁ krato smara kṛtaṁ smara
krato smara kṛtaṁ smara

Let my *prāṇa* merge with the universal all-pervading *prāṇa*, let the body be burnt by fire and reduced to ashes. Now, O intelligence! Remember, please remember all that has been done, remember all that has been done.

Commentary:

The text expresses someone's last words, but it is not necessarily referring to a physical death. At first glance, it appears to be a prayer a religious person might make on their deathbed. In fact, it is uttered by a very advanced spiritual aspirant just prior to enlightenment, the ego's death. This verse describes awakening to the reality of the eternal union of the individual and the universal, that is, the disappearance all that is personal as it unites with the Whole.

The text reflects the soul's state of consciousness of as it enters *samādhi*. In reality, the sage is sharing a valuable testimony of the ego's death. These words come from a dual perspective in the final stages of the retro-evolutionary process. They are a farewell to oneself: a simultaneous death and rebirth. It is the agony of dying on the relative plane to be reborn in the absolute, dying in time to be resurrected in eternity. It is the direct account of a spark at the moment it merges into the bonfire. It is dying as someone to live in everyone as a presence. It is dying as something in order to become nothing and live in everything. It is dying as a human to be reborn as divinity. It is ceasing to be somewhere in order to become absolute beingness.

"Let my *prāṇa* merge with the universal all-pervading *prāṇa*..."

In various Upanishadic texts, we can see that *prāṇā* is not only considered to be vital energy, but also Brahman, the Self, or consciousness:

स एष इह प्रविष्ट आ नखाग्रेभ्यः, यथा क्षुरः क्षुरधानेऽवहितः स्यात्, विश्वम्भरो वा विश्वम्भरकुलाये; तं न पश्यन्ति । अकृत्स्नो हि सः, प्राणन्नेव णो नाम भवति, वदन् वाक्, पश्यंश्चक्षुः, शृण्वन् श्रोत्रम्, मन्वानो मनः; तान्यस्यैतानि कर्मनामान्येव ।

sa eṣa iha praviṣṭa ā nakhāgrebhyaḥ, yathā kṣuraḥ kṣura-dhāne 'vahitaḥ syāt, viśvambharo vā viśvambhara-kulāye; taṁ na paśyanti akṛtsno hi saḥ, prāṇann eva prāṇo nāma bhavati, vadan vāk, paśyaṁś-cakṣuḥ, śṛṇvan śrotram, manvāno manaḥ; tāny asyaitāni karma-nāmāny eva.

This Self has entered into these bodies up to the tip of the nails as a razor may be put in its case, or as fire, which sustains the world, may be in its source. People do not see it, for (viewed in its aspects) it is incomplete. When it does the function of living, it is called the vital force; when it speaks, the organ of speech; when it sees, the eye; when it hears, the ear; and when it thinks, the mind. These are merely its names according to functions.
(*Bṛhad-āraṇyaka Upanishad*, 1.4.7)

Indra, the Lord of the gods, instructed Pratardana on how to endow human beings with what is most beneficial. Indra defined *prāṇā* in the following way:

स एष प्राण एव प्रज्ञात्मानन्दोऽजरोऽमृतः ।

sa eṣa prāṇa eva prajñātmānando 'jaro 'mṛtaḥ.

This *prāṇa* is consciousness; it is eternal bliss without death.

(*Kauṣitaki-brāmaṇa Upanishad*, 3.8)

The text refers to the yoga, or "union," of individual consciousness with the all-pervading universal consciousness. In leaping from partiality to wholeness, an existential change occurs. The "I" relaxes and fades into the infinite ocean of consciousness, like a wave dissolving into the sea. If a wave relaxes, it simply returns to its oceanic origin. The separate identity, the sense of being "the doer" of what happens to us, evaporates. As it submerges into ultimate reality, the illusory sense of a separate personality disappears.

However, any effort to conceptualize the quantum leap from mind to non-mind is ridiculous and puerile. It is impossible for a frog that only knows its pond to imagine the vast ocean. The human mind is incapable of conceiving a living subjectivity devoid of limits and boundaries, that is, an existence that palpitates and lives through us as it experiences itself. The objective mind is unable to imagine what is beyond objectivity.

The great disciple of the Baal Shem Tov, Dov Ber ben Avraham of Mezeritch, called the Maggid of Mezeritch (who died in 1772), said that the path of the spirit entails a transformation of the *ani*, or "I," into *ain*, or "nothing." It is the recognition of consciousness.

הַקָּבָּ"ה בְּרָא אֶת הָעוֹלָם יֵשׁ מֵאַיִן, וְהַצַּדִּיקִים עוֹשִׂים בְּמַעֲשֵׂיהֶם אַיִ"ן מִיֵּ"שׁ. כְּמוֹ מַעֲשֵׂה הַקָּרְבָּנוֹת, שֶׁהַבְּהֵמָה הִיא יֵשׁ, מַעֲשֵׂה גַּשְׁמִי, וְהַצַּדִּיקִים מְקָרְבִין אוֹתָהּ אֶל הַקְּדֻשָּׁה וְנַעֲשֶׂה אַיִן רוּחָנִי. נִמְצָא כִּי מִתְּחִלָּה הָיָה אַיִ"ן וּלְבַסּוֹף אַיִ"ן. וְזֶהוּ אֲנִ"י אוֹתִיּוֹת אַיִ"ן, כִּי מֵאֲנִ"י שֶׁהוּא עֲשִׂיָּה נַעֲשֶׂה אַיִ"ן.
(המגיד ממעזריטש, אור תורה, פרשת אמור, ק"כ)

The Holy One, blessed be He, created the world 'ex nihilo' ('something from nothing' or 'existence from inexistence') and the saints in their actions transform something into nothing. As in the sacrificial act, the beast is 'something,' material creation, and the saints bring it closer to divinity, so it becomes spiritual 'nothing'. Thus, you find that in the beginning it was nothing and at the end nothing. And this explains why the word ANI ('I') has the same letters as the word AIN ('nothingness'), for ANI ('I'), which is related to the world of action, becomes AIN ('nothingness'). (The Maggid of Mezeritch, *Or Torah*, Emor, 120)

"Let the body be burnt by fire and reduced to ashes."

Fire occupies a central place in Hindu, Buddhist, and

Jain liturgy. It is required for the main ceremonies and in temples, is offered daily to deities. Rituals that include offerings made to a sacred fire are called *homa*, though many call them *yajña*. The ashes that remain after *homa* are called *vibhūti* and are considered sacred. At the end of the ritual, participants often apply the ashes to their foreheads, according to the markings of their sects. In many sacred places in India and Nepal, there are *sādhus* whose bodies are covered in sacred ashes, especially *śāivas*.

The clothing of renounced Hindu monks is usually orange. This is the color of fire, which symbolizes the essence of the cosmic manifestation. Fire is a great equalizer, because after passing through the flames, everything turns to ashes equally. Whether a poor person or a millionaire, a thief or a judge, a criminal or a saint, an atheist or a religious person, when burned in fire, the same substance remains: ashes. If we burn banknotes or newspaper, we will get exactly the same ashes. When the movie ends, regardless of whether it was a drama or a comedy, only the imperturbable screen remains. Similarly, when we burn the pursuit of sensory pleasure in the flames of wisdom, what remains is Brahman, the one consciousness.

"Now, O intelligence!"

Here, the sage addresses his intelligence and requests *krato smara kṛtaṁ smara*, or "remember everything done."

In the Bhagavad Gita, Kṛṣṇa says that he himself is the ritual.

अहं क्रतुरहं यज्ञः स्वधाहमहमौषधम् ।
मन्त्रोऽहमहमेवाज्यमहमग्निरहं हुतम् ॥

ahaṁ kratur ahaṁ yajñaḥ
svadhāham aham auṣadham
mantro 'ham aham evājyam
aham agnir ahaṁ hutam

> But I am the sacrifice, the offering to the ancestors, the healing herb, the transcendental chant. I am the butter and the fire and the offering.
>
> (Bhagavad Gita, 9.16)

Krato comes from *kratu*, which means, among other connotations, "sacrifice, intelligence, and enlightenment." *Kṛta* means "what has been done" and refers to both the teachings and efforts to live by them. These teachings consist of forgetting what we think we are and remembering what we really are, to forget the separate "I" and remember consciousness, to forget the illusory separation and remember the Self. Kṛṣṇa refers to our highest ideal:

अन्तकाले च मामेव स्मरन्मुक्त्वा कलेवरम् ।
यः प्रयाति स मद्भावं याति नास्त्यत्र संशयः ॥

anta-kāle ca mām eva
smaran muktvā kalevaram
yaḥ prayāti sa mad-bhāvaṁ
yāti nāsty atra saṁśayaḥ

And whoever certainly at the end of life leaves the body remembering me alone, at once attains my nature. Of this there is no doubt.

(Bhagavad Gita, 8.5)

Anta-kāle ca mām eva means "certainly, at the end of life." The instance before death or enlightenment cannot be an isolated moment that is different from the rest of a yogi's life. Focusing on the Absolute is the consequence of a life dedicated to spiritual cultivation. If we are robbed on the street, it is not the time to start practicing karate. Once we are on our deathbed, it is too late to enroll in a meditation course. Kṛṣṇa advises arriving at the time of death by "remembering me alone."

Some may think that the Gita suggests focusing on the specific individual called Kṛṣṇa. When those who identify with the mind–body complex hear the master say "I" or "me," they mistakenly think the master is referring to himself as a person.

Most people use the word "I" to refer to a dream, but some use the same term to refer to reality. While by saying "me" many indicate an illusion, others use the same expression point to eternity. Behind the ego's "I" lies objective reality, but behind the "I" of those who see lies the Whole. Behind the "me" of the awakened one resides a presence that is a shadow of existence. Jesus said: "I am the way, the Truth, and the life. No one comes to the Father except through me." (John, 14:6). His followers infer that the person called Jesus is the way, the Truth, and the life. Consequently, they believed that no one could approach God unless he does so exclusively through Jesus. Unfortunately, this phenomenon has often occurred in the history of humankind, giving birth to organized religion and fanaticism. What happened with Jesus and Kṛṣṇa also happened with Muhammad, Buddha, Guru Nanak, Mahavira, Caitanya, and many others. This is followed by "the swing of the egoic phenomenon," that is, the same fanatics who idolize a master end up crucifying him. Retroprogressive Yoga is an invitation to recognize the reality of the "me." This is how Kṛṣṇa refers to himself in the Bhagavad Gita:

अहं सर्वस्य प्रभवो मत्तः सर्वं प्रवर्तते ।
इति मत्वा भजन्ते मां बुधा भावसमन्विताः ॥

ahaṁ sarvasya prabhavo
mattaḥ sarvaṁ pravartate
iti matvā bhajante māṁ
budhā bhāva-samanvitāḥ

I am the source of all spiritual and material worlds. Everything emanates from me. The wise who know this perfectly engage in my devotional

> service and worship me with all their hearts.
>
> (Bhagavad Gita, 10.8)

If we ask someone, "who are you?" they will most likely answer with their name, profession, nationality, or belief: James, Charles, Hindu, Arab, Russian, physician, or teacher. Our ignorance limits self-perception to a superficial and purely corporeal concept. When they say "I," almost everyone means the body–mind complex. On the contrary, sages refer to eternal and infinite consciousness. Jesus said, "I and the Father are one." (John, 10:30). On one occasion, a disciple of Jesus asked him this:

> Philip said, "Lord, show us the Father and that will be enough for us." Jesus answered: "Don't you know me, Philip, even after I have been among you such a long time? Anyone who has seen me has seen the Father. How can you say, 'Show us the Father'? Don't you believe that I am in the Father, and that the Father is in me? The words I say to you, I do not speak on my own authority. Rather, it is the Father, living in me, who is doing his work."
>
> (New Testament, John, 14:8–10)

Kṛṣṇa proposes a constant focus on the Self.

तस्मात्सर्वेषु कालेषु मामनुस्मर युध्य च ।
मय्यर्पितमनोबुद्धिर्मामेवैष्यस्यसंशयः ॥

tasmāt sarveṣu kāleṣu
mām anusmara yudhya ca
mayy arpita-mano-buddhir
mām evaiṣyasy asaṁśayaḥ

> Therefore, always remember me and also do your duty of fighting the war. With mind and intellect surrendered to me, you will definitely attain me; of this, there is no doubt.
>
> (Bhagavad Gita, 8.7)

Kṛṣṇa understands his disciple's mind and knows that delaying is a human trait. If Kṛṣṇa had told him from the very beginning that he must constantly remember him for the rest of his life, Arjuna would have postponed this. Obviously, it is not a good idea to wait until death, whether of the body or the ego. Therefore, the master reverses the guidance. First, he talks about the importance of focusing at the time of death. Since it can be very difficult, he then recommends focusing on him at all times of life, so at the end, we are experts and not beginners.

The Hebrew revelation uses the word *teshuvah*, meaning "return or go back," to refer to a retroprogressive process of returning to the original source, to our divine origin. The path of the Torah does not use terms such as "becoming religious" or "repenting of sins" but simply "returning or coming back." Anyone who ventures in search of Truth is called *baal teshuvah*, or "a master of the return." This term refers not only to the acceptance of a faith, but to an authentic transformation. To return to where we truly belong or to return to ourselves. This term has inspired me to baptize my teachings Retroprogressive Yoga.

In *Pirkei Avot*, we read the words of the great sage Rabbi Eliezer:

וְשׁוּב יוֹם אֶחָד לִפְנֵי מִיתָתְךָ.

(פרקי אבות ב', י')

And return one day before your death.

(*Pirkei Avot*, 2.10)

There is a *midrash agadah* from the time of the second temple that comments on this verse. *Midrashei agadah* are part of the oral Torah; they are teachings about the passages and laws of the Torah that were passed down as stories. There are *midrashim* to the Talmud, texts before and after the Talmud, both in different compilations, and in all rabbinic literature.

תְּנַן הָתָם, רַבִּי אֱלִיעֶזֶר אוֹמֵר: שׁוּב יוֹם אֶחָד לִפְנֵי מִיתָתְךָ. שָׁאֲלוּ תַּלְמִידָיו אֶת רַבִּי אֱלִיעֶזֶר: וְכִי אָדָם יוֹדֵעַ אֵיזֶהוּ יוֹם יָמוּת? אָמַר לָהֶן: וְכָל שֶׁכֵּן, יָשׁוּב הַיּוֹם, שֶׁמָּא יָמוּת לְמָחָר, וְנִמְצָא כָּל יָמָיו בִּתְשׁוּבָה. וְאַף שְׁלֹמֹה אָמַר בְּחָכְמָתוֹ (קהלת ט', ח'): "בְּכָל עֵת יִהְיוּ בְגָדֶיךָ לְבָנִים וְשֶׁמֶן עַל רֹאשְׁךָ אַל יֶחְסָר".

(תלמוד בבלי, שבת, קנ"ג א')

We learned there in a *Mishnah* that Rabbi Eliezer says: "Return one day before your death." Rabbi Eliezer's disciples questioned him: "Do any of us know the day we will die?" Rabbi Eliezer answered: "All the more so, we should return today lest we will die tomorrow; acting this way, we will spend all our days in a state of return (*teshuvah*)." And King Solomon also said in his wisdom: "At all times your clothes should be white, and oil shall not be absent from upon your head" (Ecclesiastes 9:8).

(*Talmud Bavli*, *Shabbat*, 153:1)

The Rambam says that since we do not know when we will die, we should continually return to the source.

לְעוֹלָם יִרְאֶה אָדָם עַצְמוֹ כְּאִלּוּ הוּא נוֹטֶה לָמוּת וְשֶׁמָּא יָמוּת בִּשְׁעָתוֹ וְנִמְצָא עוֹמֵד בְּחֶטְאוֹ. לְפִיכָךְ יָשׁוּב מֵחֲטָאָיו מִיָּד וְלֹא יֵאָמֵר כְּשֶׁאַזְקִין אָשׁוּב שֶׁמָּא יָמוּת טֶרֶם שֶׁיַּזְקִין. הוּא שֶׁשְּׁלֹמֹה אָמַר בְּחָכְמָתוֹ (קהלת ט', ח') "בְּכָל עֵת יִהְיוּ בְגָדֶיךָ לְבָנִים".

(רמב"ם, משנה תורה, הלכות תשובה, פרק ז', הלכה ב')

We should always think that we are leaning toward death, with the possibility that we might die at any time, and death may catch us before we've returned. Therefore, we should always return immediately. We should not say: "When I will grow older, I will return," for perhaps we will die before we grow older. This was implied by the

> wise advice given by King Solomon (Ecclesiastes, 9:8): "At all times, your clothes should be white." (Maimonides, *Mishneh Torah*, *Hilchot Teshuvah*, 7.2)

In fact, retroprogression is an intense way of life, as if every moment were the last.

"... Remember, please remember all that has been done."

This Upanishadic verse shows us a sage's prayer at the time of a strange and mysterious death, one that is voluntary and desired. This death does not mark the end of life, but the beginning of true living. It is a death that leads to a rebirth. With each awakening, a dream dies, which is sometimes a nightmare. With each dawn, a night dies. With each reunion, loneliness perishes.

This outcome is symbolic, because it is not the end of something that has existed. It is only the dismantling of an idea, a theory, a fantasy, a daydream, and maybe a great illusion. It is the end of an "I" that struggled without ever really coming or going, just as the Buddha explains to his disciple Subhūti:

> तद्यथाकाशे -
> तारका तिमिरं दीपो मायावश्याय बुद्बुदम् ।
> स्वप्नं च विद्युदभ्रं च एवं द्रष्टव्य संस्कृतम् ॥
> तथा प्रकाशयेत्, तेनोच्यते संप्रकाशयेदिति ॥

tad yathākāśe-
tārakā timiraṁ dīpo
māyā-vaśyāya budbudam
svapnaṁ ca vidyud abhraṁ ca
evaṁ draṣṭavya saṁskṛtam
tathā prakāśayet, tenocyate saṁprakāśayed iti

> In this way you shall conceive of this entire ephemeral world: As a star at dawn, a bubble in a torrent, a flash of lightning in a summer cloud, a flickering flame, a phantom, a dream.
>
> (*The Diamond Sūtra*, *sūtra* 32)

Science, philosophy, and mysticism agree that diversity perceived as an empirical reality arises from a single, essential origin.

According to science, objective multiplicity comes from a quantum fluctuation that materialized by amplifying itself. The Big Bang theory states that the entire universe arose from a single particle of pure energy with extreme density and high temperature.

For Greek philosophers, as well as for the sages of classical India, time was cyclical. They sought a single principle that everything emerged from and is heading toward. They strove to deduce the exodus, or *exitus* in Latin, a single principle from which everything leaves and to which all returns, *nostos* in Greek and *reditus* in Latin. The *Vedānta Sūtra* calls it Brahman, saying that it is *janmādyasya yataḥ*, or "that from which everything proceeds, is sustained, and finally dissolves."

Thales of Miletus proposed this principle was water. Heraclitus used the metaphor of fire to refer to *logos*. Parmenides argued that being is the principle of all universality. Anaximenes said it was air and explained it with a famous comparison to the soul: just as the human soul is air, which provides cohesion, the origin is a breath or divine air from the cosmic soul, the *nous*, which contains the universe. Interestingly, something similar is found in the Hebrew revelation:

> וַיִּיצֶר ה' אֱלֹקִים אֶת הָאָדָם עָפָר מִן הָאֲדָמָה וַיִּפַּח בְּאַפָּיו נִשְׁמַת חַיִּים וַיְהִי הָאָדָם לְנֶפֶשׁ חַיָּה.
> (בראשית ב', ז')

> Then the Lord God formed man (*Adam*) of the dust of the ground (*Adamah*) and blew into his nostrils the breath of life; and man became a living soul.
> (Genesis, 2:7)

Finally, mysticism also says that in the beginning, there was plenitude. It refers to the primordial unity, or the wholeness of consciousness. From its rupture, multiplicity emerges. In Greek, it is called *pleroma,* from the verb *pléroó* meaning "to make full." To understand the rupture of the *pleroma*, we must turn to the first few chapters of Hegel's *Phenomenology of Spirit*.

Aristotle said that only God exists and his only activity is to think thoughts. That is, God is the thought that thinks itself. And it is by thinking itself that absolute non-duality becomes diversified. By thinking itself, unity becomes plurality: subject and object, thinker and thought. It means being both subject and object at the same time. As a thought thinking itself, God is both unity and duality: simultaneous undifferentiation and differentiation. Just like Śrī Caitanya Mahāprabhu's brilliant Gauḍīya Vaiṣṇava concept of *acintya-bheda-abheda tattva*, or "inconceivable one and simultaneously different." Kṛṣṇadāsa Kavirāja Gosvāmī describes this concept in Bengali:

রাধাকৃষ্ণ এক আত্মা, দুই দেহ ধরি' ।
অন্যোন্যে বিলসে রস আস্বাদন করি' ॥

rādhā-kṛṣṇa eka ātmā, dui deha dhari'
anyonye vilase rasa āsvādana kari'

Rādhā and Kṛṣṇa are one and the same, but they have assumed two bodies. Thus, they enjoy each other, tasting the mellows of love.
(*Śrī Caitanya-caritāmṛta*, "*Ādi-līlā*," 4.56)

Before the appearance of logos, classical cosmogonies described the relationship between unity and division, or separation and return to the source, with retroprogressive movement. Throughout the world's mythology, this relationship is expressed in different narratives that mention the dismemberment of a divine being as the origin of the universe. In the Mesopotamian creation myth *Enuma Elish*, also known as "The Seven Tablets of Creation," Marduk creates the heavens and the earth from the corpse of Tiamat. Marduk, the god of wisdom, after being praised for his victory and consulting Ea, creates humans from clay kneaded with the blood of the demon Kingu, who advised Tiamat to fight. Human beings were created to help the gods in their eternal function of maintaining order and avoiding chaos.

> Ea created humankind / On whom he imposed the service of the gods, and set the gods free.
>
> (Tablet VI.33–34)

Empirical reality is understood as the dismemberment of a non-dual totality, which must come with the search for the Whole. Plato calls this "reuniting the dispersed" in *The Banquet*.

> So ancient is the desire of one another which is implanted in us, reuniting our original nature, making one of two, and healing the state of man. Each of us when separated, having one side only, like a flat fish, is but the indenture of a man, and he is always looking for his other half.

Different cosmogonies all describe a segmentation of the divine non-dual, or an original paradise, and a return to the source.

The ancient Egyptians tried to explain the origin of

the universe with a complex cosmogony. The myth of Isis and Osiris contains the essence of Egyptian spirituality. Isis recomposes the body of Osiris that was torn to pieces by his brother Set.

The primitive religious experience of the Greeks grew out of the cult of Dionysus, who planted the seed of accepting the soul's eternity and divinity. From these two beliefs, Greek mysticism was born, which did not organize into a formal religion but attracted small groups of followers. Their mysticism influenced some philosophical schools, which shared with the world the reunion of the eternal soul and divinity. The latter reminds us of the Sanskrit term *yoga*, or "union" and *religion*, coming from the Latin *religio* composed of the prefix *re*, the verb *ligare*, or "to bind," and the suffix *ion*, or "action and effect of binding or tying strongly with God."

Greek mysticism aimed to shorten the distance, inherited from Homeric religion, between humans and gods. With this purpose, rituals with dances were performed in search of altered states of consciousness that would free the soul from its physical limitations and connect it to the desired deity. Those who achieved these states were called *enthoi*. For achieving altered states of consciousness, they were considered prophets and lovers that deserved respect. The word enthusiasm comes from the Greek *enthousiasmos*, a term that etymologically means "divine possession." The Greek noun is formed from the preposition *en* and the noun *theos*, or "God." Therefore, those who experience enthusiasm are possessed by a god who manifests through them.

The ancient Greeks attributed lightning, stars, and the moon to the gods. We are told that Thales of Miletus transformed these myths to *logos*, giving birth to philosophy. This revolutionary change reassessed our relationship with the universe. Henceforth, empirical reality was explained in terms of natural objects and phenomena.

In the New Testament (Revelation, 13:8), we find the phrase "the Lamb who was slain." Christianity believes that Jesus was the lamb who was sacrificed before the creation of the universe, which made it possible for everyone to have eternal life.

> He was chosen before the creation of the world,
> but was revealed in these last times for your sake.
> (New Testament, 1 Peter, 1:20)

St. Paul expresses the search for the return to the non-dual origin:

> When he has done this, then the Son himself will be made subject to him who put everything under him, so that God may be all in all.
> (1 Corinthians, 15:28)

"...remember all that has been done."

We have created an image of ourselves that we live by. We call it "I" and think of it as the "doer" of our actions. We believe that this imaginary entity is permanent, controlling, and has free will. This image is subject to human conditioning that is made up of our family, traditions, nationality, culture, and profession. It encompasses our past experiences, our interpretations of them, our inherited tendencies and habits, our triumphs and defeats, and our position in society.

The imaginary "I-doer" is like a computer's hard drive that acts repetitively and unconsciously. Completely lacking creativity, nothing original can emerge from it. It is not a real entity, but an imaginary, temporary, and insubstantial one. It is a mental creation intended to perpetuate its own existence and defend its presumed continuity. If the "I" were inside of me, then I would be outside of my "I." As important as the "doer" may seem, it is insignificant, just another drop in the ocean of life. It is a mental contraction that adds tension to activity; in its absence, action flows and existence expresses itself through us.

In his final moments, the sage turns to his intelligence, asking it to remember what has been done. Whether it is the death of a body or an ego, it is important to remember all that has been done to attain the unattainable and to remember the futility of our efforts to be what we have always been.

According to ancient Vedantic wisdom, it is of paramount importance that we transcend this "I–doer," or egoic phenomenon. Beginners often ask who transcends it. Although it might seem odd, the answer is no one. An independent "I–doer" would require a duality of subject and object, a doer and a deed. But in reality, only the Self, or non-dual consciousness, exists.

Moreover, any effort to transcend the "I–doer" would be another deed. But no action coming from the ego will be able to transcend it. Just as we cannot lift ourselves up by pulling our belt up, we cannot transcend the ego with egoic activity. It is impossible for the mind to go beyond the mind. Transcendence will only come with the recognition that the separation between subject and object is imaginary.

The separate "I–doer" is completely illusory. Only consciousness exists, therefore, we do not *do* but we *are* action. If we observe the body–mind complex, we will notice that when we want a glass of water it is enough for us to want it and we find ourselves drinking it. There is no need to command a hand or foot to move. The body moves involuntarily before choosing to do so. That is, consciousness does not desire, decide, or choose, but it is what is desired, decided, or chosen. The last step of the retroprogressive path is a quantum leap from being a doer to being a witness. Since this witness could be considered "someone," it would be better to describe it as a jump to witnessing or observing.

The sage addresses his intelligence: "Remember, please remember all that has been done." At this point, it is important to remember that realization is not obtained because of what we have done. Through action, it is impossible to reach that high. The efforts of an independent "I" cannot bring us an inch closer to recognizing consciousness. If you do not remember everything you have done, this last step will be taken with the ego, so it will perpetuate the subject–object duality.

There is a radical difference between 1) identifying with the action of thinking, feeling, and perceiving and 2) observing thoughts, emotions, sensations, and perceptions. In the former, we mistakenly consider ourselves to be doers, while in the latter we only observe what happens. Identifying with thoughts, sensations, or perceptions leads us to ascribe these activities to ourselves, entangling us in the position of thinker, feeler, or perceiver. All mental activity is based on the idea of a thinker. However, from observation, we distance ourselves from such activity, which is objectified as an occurrence and observed until it disappears. Kṛṣṇa says:

यत्करोषि यदश्नासि यज्जुहोषि ददासि यत् ।
यत्तपस्यसि कौन्तेय तत्कुरुष्व मदर्पणम् ॥

yat karoṣi yad aśnāsi
yaj juhoṣi dadāsi yat
yat tapasyasi kaunteya
tat kuruṣva mad-arpaṇam

Whatever you do, whatever you eat, whatever you offer or give away, and whatever austerities you perform – do that, O son of Kuntī, as an offering to me.

(Bhagavad Gita, 9.27)

The role of the doer arises from focusing on repetitive activity rather than on what is actually happening. When consciousness is directed toward automatic activity instead of actual occurrences, we fall into the role of the doer. The mind objectifies this role by gradually accepting each situation as natural, spontaneous, and authentic. The "I-doer" personalizes impersonal situations and interprets them as the result of its doing.

The retroprogressive *teshuvah* path is an invitation to renounce the activity of a doer in order to notice occurrences from the void. The return to the origin, to what we really are, does not mean performing an action in the ordinary sense of the phrase. Instead, it is a return to what is impossible to abandon. Retroprogressive action is both progress and return at the same time. What is needed is relaxation and inaction. No activity executed by a doer leads to meditative inaction. Effortless action is a flow of consciousness.

When walking, renounce the idea that "I walk." When drinking, renounce the idea that "I drink." When speaking, do not think of yourself as the speaker. When eating, do not think of yourself as the eater. The independent doer "I" is completely unnecessary to live. It does not matter who acts or performs the action, but that which cognizes it, knows it, and observes it. In reality, our authentic nature is the knower of experience. You are not the doer. It is consciousness, or Kṛṣṇa, that acts through you.

MANTRA 18

अग्ने नय सुपथा राये अस्मान्
विश्वानि देव वयुनानि विद्वान् ।
युयोध्यस्मज्जुहुराणमेनो
भूयिष्ठां ते नमउक्तिं विधेम ॥

agne naya supathā rāye asmān
viśvāni deva vayunāni vidvān
yuyodhy asmaj juhurāṇam eno
bhūyiṣṭhāṁ te nama-uktiṁ vidhema

O Agni, Lord of the sacrificial fire! Guide us to wealth on the right path, O knower of our activities! Liberate us from the attraction to sin; we offer you our most humble and respectful reverences.

Commentary:

"O Agni, Lord of the sacrificial fire!"

According to the sacred scriptures of *Sanātana-dharma*, each element in nature is ruled by a specific deity. Agni presides over fire, or *tejas*. Due to the importance of fire in many rituals in the Vedic tradition, Agni is a central deity. As Vedic chanting developed over time, Agni became the deity with the most hymns. His role is to accept offerings from devotees and deliver them to their celestial recipients. He also leads the invoked gods to their respective ceremonies. Because of his function as an intermediary between earth and the heaven, Agni is considered to be the mouth of the gods and goddesses. The *Sanātana-dharma* considers him to be the mediator par excellence between human beings and the gods because of his presence on three different levels: on earth as fire, in the atmosphere as lightning, and in the sky as the sun. Other forms of fire associated with Agni include the fire of sacrificial rituals, the fire of funeral pyres, and the digestive fire that operates inside our bodies.

The sage Bhṛgu conceived of the purifying capacity of the fire of Agni. Few elements are as destructive and purifying as fire. On one hand, Śiva's fire destroys the universe, but on the other, Agni's fire cleanses and purifies sinful human reactions. Because of its purifying properties, it is invoked on the funeral pyre when corpses are cremated. Agni also leads the souls of the departed to Lord Yamarāja, the god of death. He and his twin brother Indra, the god of the heavens and rains, and Sūrya, the sun god, occupy a prominent place as the Vedic triad. The *Mahābhārata* says that because of their indulgence in over-consuming offerings, this triad was displaced in the post-Vedic or Puranic era.

Agni is the witness to the activities of every human being. Although he is immortal, he agrees to reside among mortals and protect monarchs and their families. He resides in every household to do one of three things: provide domestic support (*gārhapatyāgni*), invite and welcome (*āhavanīyāgni*), or protect against evil (*dakṣiṇāgni*). Even today, he is invoked by faithful Hindus who ask for blessings on solemn occasions. His presence is still felt in Hindu tradition when lighting a lamp at a birth celebration, at *pūjā*, at marriages when the bride and groom circle the fire seven times, and at cremation after death.

According to the *Atharva Veda,* Agni removes the soul of the deceased from the burning pyre so it can be reborn in the next life. The oldest Vedic texts point out that the cosmic manifestation began with Prajāpati or Brahman, such as section 6.1 of the *Kāṭhaka Saṁhitā* and section 1.8.1 of the *Maitrāyaṇī Saṁhitā*. Agni emerged from the forehead of Prajāpati. Along with the manifestation of Agni came light, and from light, day and night. According to these *Saṁhitās*, Agni is Brahman. In later Vedic texts, there is a complex mythology of the origins of Agni, explained in section 2.1.2 of the *Taittirīya*

Brāhmaṇa and sections 2.2.3–4 of the *Śatapatha Brāhmaṇa*. His name can vary: Vahni (the one who receives the *homa*, or "the burnt sacrifice"), Vītihotra (the one who sanctifies the worshipper), Dhanañjaya (the conqueror of wealth), Jīvānala (the one who burns), Dhūmaketu (the one whose sign is smoke), Chāga-ratha (the one who rides on a ram), and Sapta-jihvā (the one who has seven tongues), among others.

In Puranic literature and in important epic poems, he is mentioned as being born from the face of the Cosmic Being or Virāṭ Puruṣa. In other writings, he appears as the son of Pṛthivī, the Earth goddess, and Pitar, or Father god. Other sources say he is the son of the gods Aditi and Kaśyapa. His consorts, or *śaktis*, are Svāhā and Svadhā. Agni is the father of the god of war, Skanda or Kārtikeya. In the *Mahābhārata*, Agni grows weary from consuming too many offerings. In order to regain his energy, he tries to consume the Khandava forest. Indra tries to stop him, but in the end, Agni manages to confuse Indra with the help of Kṛṣṇa and Arjuna, and achieves his goal.

In the Rig Veda, Indra and the other gods are called upon to destroy their enemies, the flesh-eating *rākṣasas* or *kravyāds*. Although Agni was also a *kravyād*, he destroys them. In the *Rāmāyaṇa*, we read that Agni incarnated as Nīla to help Lord Rāmacandra.

The iconography of Agni varies by region. In the *Āgamas*, he is depicted as an old man with a fiery red body, two heads, six eyes, three legs, and seven pairs of arms. One of his names is Sapta-jihvā, or "possessor of seven tongues," which he uses to relish butter that he drinks from sacrifices. His body expels seven flames or luminous rays. His two heads with two faces represent his destructive and benevolent powers. He travels riding a goat or a chariot pulled by goats or parrots.

In fact, the veneration of fire and the sun has characterized almost all peoples throughout history. In most traditions and cultures, rituals and legends have been recorded in paintings and writings that document their beliefs. Religions, esotericism, alchemy, and astrology have given great importance to fire and the sun in relation to the human being. From the earliest times of mankind, fire has been a sign of salvation, protection, and nourishment.

וְנָתְנוּ בְּנֵי אַהֲרֹן הַכֹּהֵן אֵשׁ עַל־הַמִּזְבֵּחַ וְעָרְכוּ עֵצִים עַל־הָאֵשׁ.
וְעָרְכוּ בְּנֵי אַהֲרֹן הַכֹּהֲנִים אֵת הַנְּתָחִים אֶת־הָרֹאשׁ וְאֶת־הַפָּדֶר
עַל־הָעֵצִים אֲשֶׁר עַל־הָאֵשׁ אֲשֶׁר עַל־הַמִּזְבֵּחַ.
(ויקרא א', ז'-ח')

The sons of Aaron the priest shall put fire on the altar and lay out wood upon the fire; and Aaron's sons, the priests, shall lay out the sections, with the head and the fat, on the wood that is on the fire upon the altar.

(Leviticus, 1:7–8)

"...we offer you our most humble and respectful reverences."

This mantra is a devotional prayer made by the sage with respect and veneration. It is addressed to a personal aspect of divinity, suggesting harmony between bhakti and *jñāna*. Many mistakenly believe that Advaita Vedanta conflicts with devotion. They believe that worshipping God is incompatible with a non-dualistic perspective. If only Brahman is real, the world is illusory, and the individual soul is Brahman, then we would be worshipping ourselves. At first glance, it seems as ridiculous as begging for alms from a millionaire when we ourselves are that millionaire. Without experiencing it, the worshipper–worshipped relationship may seem dishonest. To delve deeper into the issue of devotion, which is so central to the retroprogressive process, we must explore the philosophical reasons for worship. Worshipping a personal God and realizing non-dualism happen at different levels of reality. Although absolute reality is all one, Advaita Vedanta proposes three levels of reality: real, unreal, and non-real. What is true always exists, and what is false never existed. The Truth is, was, and will never cease to be. As this verse states:

नासतो विद्यते भावो नाभावो विद्यते सतः ।
उभयोरपि दृष्टोऽन्तस्त्वनयोस्तत्त्वदर्शिभिः ॥

nāsato vidyate bhāvo
nābhāvo vidyate sataḥ
ubhayor api dṛṣṭo 'ntas
tv anayos tattva-darśibhiḥ

The seers of the Truth have concluded that what is nonexistent does not endure and what is eternal does not change. This they have concluded by studying the nature of both.

(Bhagavad Gita, 2.16)

Śaṅkara offers a brilliant explanation of the phenomenon of the world and its relation to ultimate reality. In his writings, he mentions three orders or levels of reality: absolute reality (*pāramārthika*), relative reality (*vyāvahārika*), and illusory reality (*prātibhāsika*), which he distinguishes from non-existence (*alīka*).

यद्वा त्रिविधं सत्त्वम् - पारमार्थिकं व्यावहारिकं प्रातिभासिकं चेति । पारमार्थिकं सत्त्वं ब्रह्मणः व्यावहारिकं सत्त्वमाकाशादेः प्रातिभासिकं सत्त्वं शुक्तिरजतादेः ।

yad vā tri-vidhaṁ sattvam- pāramārthikaṁ vyāvahārikaṁ pratibhāsikañ ceti. pāramārthikaṁ sattvaṁ brahmaṇaḥ, vyāvahārikaṁ sattvam ākāśādeḥ, prātibhāsikaṁ sattvaṁ śukti-rajatādeḥ.

[Or we may say] there are three kinds of existence: absolute, conventional, and illusory.

> Absolute existence belongs to Brahman, conventional existence to the ether, and so on, and illusory existence to the silver in nacre.
>
> (*Vedānta-paribhāṣā*, chapter 1)

Absolute reality or *pāramārthika-sattā*: This refers to Brahman, which is the only reality that exists; it is pure, immutable, and eternal. Objective phenomena are unreal superimpositions over the background of this absolute reality. From the point of view of *pāramārthika-sattā*, both relative and illusory reality are false. Differences between the two are only relevant to those who are still blinded by ignorance. Those who have realized transcendental consciousness perceive that plurality is a manifestation of a single reality. Plurality vanishes along with the disappearance of ignorance. In a state of transcendental consciousness, the absolute reality (*pāramārthika*) underlying the objective diversity of names and forms is perceived. Just as an ordinary person knows that the moon reflected in the lake is not the real moon, a realized being perceives that objects are unreal. The wise ones look at the objective world like we look at a mirror: knowing that the reality they see is only a reflection.

Relative reality or *vyāvahārika-sattā*: This is the empirical, practical, relative, and temporal reality that is based on subject–object relationships. Śaṅkara reveals in his commentary on the *Vedānta Sūtra* that *vyāvahārika-sattā* comes from the mutual superimposition of the real and the unreal, or the Self and non-Self, caused by ignorance.

Every existing phenomenon combines reality and unreality. Since *vyāvahārika-sattā* is based on time, space, and causality, it is constantly mutating. Its temporary nature differentiates it from absolute reality, which is eternal. Even though the objective world is only an empirical reality, in practical life we should relate to the world as if it were real.

Illusory reality or *prātibhāsika-sattā*: *Prātibhāsika* is only an appearance of *vyāvahārika*. It refers to the apparent reality of the illusory phenomena, such as hallucinations, mirages, dreams, and so on. This reality is accepted as real as long as the illusion lasts, but this ends when we become conscious of empirical reality (*vyāvahārika*). These illusions originate in *avidyā*, or "ignorance," and they vanish as soon as we recognize the real basis that gave rise to the illusion. The illusion dissipates only through the knowledge of essence, or *adhiṣṭhāna*.

Prātibhāsika is like the reflection of the moon in a calm and peaceful lake. Although it is only an appearance, the reflection may seem to be the moon itself. The reflection of the moon is perceptible, but the reflected moon is false. It may be very beautiful, but it is illusory. The true moon is considered real only when it is compared to its reflection.

Inexistence or *alīka*: This refers to absolute non-existence. The three levels of reality mentioned above are different from *alīka*. It is impossible to perceive *alīka* in the past, present, or future, for example, a son of a sterile woman.

For Śaṅkara, only absolute reality (*pāramārthika*) exists, whereas relative reality (*vyāvahārika*) is non-real, or *mithyā*. The objective universe is a non-real phenomenon (*mithyā*) but perceptible.

अवाच्छिन्नाश्चिदाभासस्तृतीयः स्वप्नकल्पितः।
विज्ञेयस्त्रिविधोजीवस्तत्राद्यः परमार्थिकः ॥

avācchinnaś cid-ābhāsas
tritīyaḥ svapna-kalpitaḥ
vijñeyas tri-vidho jīvas
tatrādyaḥ pāramārthikaḥ

> There are three conceptions of *jīva* (consciousness): one is limited by *prāṇa* (vital energy), one is present in the mind, and one is consciousness as imagined in dream [to have assumed the forms of humans, and so on]. The first of these is true nature.
>
> (*Dṛg-dṛṣya-viveka*, 32)

From an absolute perspective, or *pāramārthika*, Vedanta asserts that the universe is false and only Brahman is real. Everything is a single undivided consciousness, therefore, we are consciousness or Brahman itself. That is what Śaṅkarācārya is talking about in this famous phrase:

ब्रह्म सत्यं जगन्मिथ्या जीवो ब्रह्मैव नापरः।

brahma satyaṁ jagan mithyā
jīvo brahmaiva nāparaḥ

> Brahman is real. The universe is false. The *jīva* itself is Brahman: it is not different from Brahman.
>
> (*Brahma-jñānāvalī-mālā*, 20a)

Mithyā means "non-real or false." *Jagan mithyā* indicates that the universe is apparent: although it is false, it seems real. Multiplicity appears to have a separate existence. Illusion, or *māyā*, is the belief that dual experience is ultimate reality. From the non-dual perspective, it is evident that the objective universe is apparent. Even so apparent duality is not in conflict with absolute and ultimate reality.

"Brahman is reality, the world is an appearance, and you are Brahman" is true from the perspective of absolute reality. But from a dual point of view, Brahman can be identified with the body and mind and worshipped as Kṛṣṇa, or a personal God. We must clarify that Advaita Vedanta speaks only from and about absolute reality.

Clearly, by performing *pūjā* to Their Lordships Śrī Śrī Radha-Śyāmasundara, we are acting on the relative platform, or *vyāvahārika*. But worshipping Kṛṣṇa on the relative platform is not incompatible with the absoluteness of consciousness. No matter how non-dualistic we may be, we eat food, wear clothes, exercise our muscles, and converse with others. The absurdity is that we only reject dualistic practices related to God while, in relative reality, we carry out endless dualistic activities.

However, as mentioned in the *Pañcadaśī*, non-dual ultimate reality is compatible with our illusory experience of duality. The opposite would be incompatible, that is, if absolute reality were dual and our experience were non-dual.

Even though we understand that the earth is round, we can still walk on a seemingly flat surface. The roundness belongs to absolute reality; apparent flatness belongs to our relative reality. Although we know that the sky is colorless, we continue to enjoy its apparent bluish color in the morning and reddish color at sunset. Nothing can be colorless and blue at the same time, but it is possible that the sky is in fact colorless, but we perceive it as having a color. Likewise, absolute reality is non-dual, but perceived as relative reality it appears to be dual.

Retroprogressive Yoga accepts both the reality of absolute union with Kṛṣṇa and apparent separation. The difference between non-dualistic devotees and dualistic devotees of Kṛṣṇa is not existential but philosophical. The dualistic devotees see the soul and God as two eternally separate entities. On the other hand, non-dualistic devotees see themselves as localized consciousness that experience consciousness as Īśvara. Devotees and Īśvara are the same consciousness, just as the waves and the ocean are both water.

The Absolute devoid of attributes is called Nirguṇa-brahman. The same Brahman, when qualified, or covered with attributes, is known as Saguṇa-brahman or Īśvara, the personal God. Nirguṇa-brahman is the essential cause of creation, while Saguṇa-brahman is the creator. *Māyā*, or "illusion," is the inherent power of Brahman. Īśvara is Brahman perceived through *māyā* from the perspective of the perceiving subject. Names and forms are illusionary and if they are removed, the worshipper is revealed to be Brahman. Kṛṣṇa himself says this in the Bhagavad Gita:

अजोऽपि सन्नव्ययात्मा भूतानामीश्वरोऽपि सन् ।
प्रकृतिं स्वामधिष्ठाय सम्भवाम्यात्ममायया ॥

ajo 'pi sann avyayātmā
bhūtānām īśvaro 'pi san
prakṛtiṁ svām adhiṣṭhāya
sambhavāmy ātma-māyayā

> Though I am unborn and am of imperishable nature, and though I am the Lord of all beings, yet, ruling over my own nature, I take birth by my own *māyā*.
>
> (Bhagavad Gita, 4.6)

As long as both the worshipper and the worshipped maintain their garments of attributes, the dual relationship between God and devotee endures, even though both are from a single indivisible reality.

Advaitic bhakti explains that non-dual reality is

unaffected by apparent dual experience. For example, currently you, the subject, are holding a book, the object. Both are within the context of a relative reality with an apparent dual subject–object relationship. Yet non-dual absolute reality, or consciousness, is all that really is. Therefore, we can affirm that both relative and absolute reality are not in different places. There is no actual separation between what is relative and what is absolute, what is illusory and what is real, what is apparent and what is true. It is perfectly possible for our experience and absolute reality to coexist.

My personal Kṛṣṇa is Brahman itself. Non-objective absolute reality, although it is devoid of attributes, manifests before us within the context experience as qualified Kṛṣṇa. Therefore, Brahman and Kṛṣṇa are not different, nor are they separate. They are one and the same, viewed from different perspectives. This is explained by our beloved Paraṁ Guru Bhagavān Śrī Mastarāma Bābājī Mahārāja in his poem *He Ananta*:

हे अनन्त नित्यमुक्त
हे स्वरूपसुन्दर
प्रियवर परावर हे स्वरूपसुन्दर
परमपुरुष अप्रमेय हेतु हेतु हे
हे अनन्य अधिपते
नमन हे नमन हे
हे अनन्य अधिपते

he ananta! nitya-mukta!
he svarūpa-sundara
priya-vara! parā-vara!
he svarūpa-sundara

parama-puruṣa! aprameya!
hetu-hetu he!
he ananya adhipate!
namana he, namana he
he ananya adhipate!

O Infinite, eternally free
O you with beautiful form
Most beloved one, formless Brahman
O one with beautiful form
Supreme person! Unfathomable being!
Cause of the cause, O Thou who are no other than my own self, Supreme Lord,
O Prostrations
O Inseparable Supreme Lord!

Kṛṣṇa is the qualified absolute whereas Brahman is Kṛṣṇa devoid of attributes. The qualified personal God is the objectification of consciousness on the platform of experiences. In a famous verse from the Bhagavad Gita, Kṛṣṇa says:

यदा यदा हि धर्मस्य ग्लानिर्भवति भारत ।
अभ्युत्थानमधर्मस्य तदात्मानं सृजाम्यहम् ॥

yadā yadā hi dharmasya
glānir bhavati bhārata
abhyutthānam adharmasya
tadātmānaṁ sṛjāmy aham

Whenever there is a decay of righteousness, O Bharata, and a rise of unrighteousness, then I manifest myself.

(Bhagavad Gita, 4.7)

Many distinguished enlightened masters have written beautiful devotional hymns. Śaṅkarācārya, the highest exponent of the Advaita school, never saw an incompatibility between non-dual reality and a personal God. He composed poems to glorify deities, such as the *Govindāṣṭakam* dedicated to Lord Kṛṣṇa:

सत्यं ज्ञानमनन्तं नित्यमनाकाशं परमाकाशं
गोष्ठप्राङ्गणरिङ्खणलोलमनायासं परमायासम् ।
मायाकल्पितनानाकारमनाकारं भुवनाकारं
क्ष्मायानाथमनाथं प्रणमत गोविन्दं परमानन्दम् ॥

satyaṁ jñānam anantaṁ nityam anākāśaṁ paramākāśaṁ
goṣṭha-prāṅgaṇa-riṅkhaṇa-lolam anāyāsaṁ paramāyāsam
māyā-kalpita-nānākāram-anākāraṁ bhuvanākāraṁ
kṣmāyā nātham-anāthaṁ praṇamata govindaṁ paramānandam

Please bow down to Govinda, supreme bliss personified. He is the absolute Truth, as well as unlimited and eternal knowledge. Though different from the sky, He Himself is the supreme sky. Though it was with effortless ease that Hess rolled and frolicked in the courtyards of Vraja, He appeared to become tired. Though formless, He manifests in various forms fashioned by *māyā*, including the form of the universe. Though He shelters all the universes, He appears to need shelter.

मृत्स्नामत्सीहेति यशोदाताडनशैशव सन्त्रासं
व्यादितवक्त्रालोकितलोकालोकचतुर्दशलोकालिम् ।
लोकत्रयपुरमूलस्तम्भं लोकालोकमनालोकं
लोकेशं परमेशं प्रणमत गोविन्दं परमानन्दम् ॥

mṛtsnām atsīheti yaśodā-tāḍana-śaiśava santrāsaṁ
vyādita-vaktrā-lokita-lokāloka-caturdaśa-lokālim
loka-traya-pura-mūla-stambhaṁ lokālokam anālokaṁ
lokeśaṁ parameśaṁ praṇamata govindaṁ paramānandam

Please bow down to Govinda, supreme bliss personified. Though he is the supreme master of the universe, he seemed to become frightened like an ordinary infant when Mother Yaśodā chastised him. When she asked, 'are you eating mud?' He opened his mouth to prove he had not, and showed her the fourteen planetary systems, including Lokāloka Mountain. He is the supporting pillar for this citylike universe of three worlds. Though He is beyond all vision, He is the source of everyone's vision.

त्रैविष्टपरिपुवीरघ्नं क्षितिभारघ्नं भवरोगघ्नं
कैवल्यं नवनीताहारमनाहारं भुवनाहारम् ।
वैमल्यस्फुटचेतोवृत्तिविशेषाभासमनाभासं
शैवं केवलशान्तं प्रणमत गोविन्दं परमानन्दम् ॥

trai-viṣṭapa-ripu-vīra-ghnaṁ kṣiti-bhāra-ghnaṁ bhava-roga-ghnaṁ
kaivalyaṁ navanītāhāram-anāhāraṁ bhuvanāhāram
vaimalya-sphuṭa-ceto-vṛtti-viśeṣābhāsam anābhāsaṁ
śaivaṁ kevala-śāntaṁ praṇamata govindaṁ paramānandam

Please bow down to Govinda, supreme bliss personified. He relieves the earth of its burden by killing the demigods' enemies, the demons, and He grants liberation by curing the disease of materialism. Though He never needs to eat, still He eats butter, and He also devours the whole universe at the time of annihilation. Though distinct from all the shadow manifestations of this world, He manifests in the sanctified desires of a pure heart. He is most auspicious and peaceful.

गोपालं प्रभुलीलाविग्रहगोपालं कुलगोपालं
गोपीखेलनगोवर्धनधृतिलीलालालितगोपालम् ।
गोभिर्निगदितगोविन्दस्फुटनामानं बहुनामानं
गोपीगोचरदूरं प्रणमत गोविन्दं परमानन्दम् ॥

gopālaṁ prabhu-līlā-vigraha-gopālaṁ kula-gopālaṁ
gopī-khelana-govardhana-dhṛti-līlā-lālita-gopālam
gobhir nigadita-govinda-sphuṭa-nāmānaṁ bahu-nāmānaṁ
gopī-gocara-dūram praṇamata govindaṁ paramānandam

Please bow down to Govinda, supreme bliss personified. That protector of cows appeared in the form of a cowherd among the cowherds to perform his pastimes on earth, such as lifting Govardhana Hill to protect the cowherds and dallying with the cowherd damsels. Even the cows called him by the name Govinda. He has unlimited names, is distinct among the cowherd boys, and is beyond the reach of the *gopīs*' senses [when he goes to the forest during the day, or when he resides in Mathurā or Dvārakā].

गोपीमण्डलगोष्ठीभेदं भेदावस्थमभेदाभं
शश्वद्गोखुरनिर्धूतोद्गतधूलीधूसरसौभाग्यम् ।
श्रद्धाभक्तिगृहीतानन्दमचिन्त्यं चिन्तितसद्भावं
चिन्तामणिमहिमानं प्रणमत गोविन्दं परमानन्दम् ॥

gopī-maṇḍala-goṣṭhī-bhedaṁ bhedāvastham abhedābhaṁ
śaśvad go-khura-nirdhūtodgata-dhūlī-dhūsara-saubhāgyam
śraddhā-bhakti-gṛhītānandam acintyaṁ cintita-sad-bhāvaṁ
cintāmaṇi mahimānaṁ praṇamata govindaṁ paramānandam

Please bow down to Govinda, supreme bliss personified. He enters the assembly of cowherd damsels and divides them into groups for his pastimes. He is simultaneously different from and one with everything. He considers it his good fortune to be always smeared with the dust raised by the cows' hooves. He is pleased by faith and devotion. Though he is inconceivable, his pastimes are the object of meditation. He is like a transcendental touchstone.

स्नानव्याकुलयोशिद्वस्त्रमुपादायागमुपारूढं
व्यादित्सन्तीरथ दिग्वस्त्रा ह्युपुदातुमुपाकर्षन्तम् ।
निर्धूतद्वयशोकविमोहं बुद्धं बुद्धेरन्तस्थं
सत्तामात्रशरीरं प्रणमत गोविन्दं परमानन्दम् ॥

snāna-vyākula-yośid-vastram upādāyagam upārūḍhaṁ
vyāditsantīr atha dig-vastrā hy upudātum upākarṣantam
nirdhūta dvaya-śoka-vimohaṁ buddhaṁ buddher antasthaṁ
sattā-mātra-śarīraṁ praṇamata govindaṁ paramānandam

Please bow down to Govinda, supreme bliss personified. He stole the bathing damsels' clothes and climbed a tree with them, and when the naked maidens asked for their clothes back, He told them to come closer. He dispels lamentation and delusion. He is knowledge personified, realized by intelligence, and is also the personification of pure existence.

कान्तं कारणकारणमादिमनादिं कालमनाभासं

कालिन्दीगतकालियशिरसि मुहुर्नृत्यन्तं नृत्यन्तम् ।
कालं कालकलातीतं कलिताशेषं कलिदोषघ्नं
कालत्रयगतिहेतुं प्रणमत गोविन्दं परमानन्दम् ॥

kāntaṁ kāraṇa-kāraṇam ādim anādiṁ kalam anābhāsaṁ
kālindī-gata-kāliya-śirasi muhur muhuḥ sunṛtyantam
kālaṁ kāla-kalātītaṁ kalitāśeṣaṁ kali-doṣa-ghnaṁ
kāla-traya-gati-hetuṁ praṇamata govindaṁ paramānandam

Please bow down to Govinda, supreme bliss personified. He is most beautiful. He is the original cause of all causes, and he has no cause. He is free from all superimpositions of illusion. He danced wonderfully on the hoods of the Kāliya serpent in the Yamunā. Though he is time, He is beyond all divisions of time. He knows everything, he destroys the defects of Kali-yuga, and he is the source of past, present, and future.

वृन्दावनभुवि वृन्दारकगणवृन्दाराध्यं वन्देऽहं
कुन्दाभामलमन्दस्मेरसुधानन्दं सुहृदानन्दम् ।
वन्द्याशेषमहामुनिमानसवन्द्यानन्दपदद्वन्द्वं
वन्द्याशेषगुणाब्धिं प्रणमत गोविन्दं परमानन्दम् ॥

vṛndāvana-bhuvi vṛndāraka-gaṇa-vṛndārādhyaṁ vande 'haṁ
kundābhāmala-manda-smera-sudhānandaṁ suhṛd-ānandam
vandyāśeṣa-mahā-muni-mānasa-vandyānanda-pada-dvandvaṁ
vandyāśeṣa-guṇābdhiṁ praṇamata govindaṁ paramānandam

Please bow down to Govinda, supreme bliss personified. He is the reservoir of all worshipable qualities. All worshipable saintly persons worship his blissful lotus feet within their hearts. He is my worshipful Lord. All the demigods, and Śrīmatī Vṛndā Devī as well, worship him in the land of Vṛndāvana. His pure and beautiful smile emanates bliss like a *kuṇḍa* flower pouring forth nectar. He gives transcendental ecstasy to his cowherd friends.

गोविन्दाष्टकमेतदधीते गोविन्दार्पितचेता यो
गोविन्दाच्युत माधव विष्णो गोकुलनायक कृष्णेति ।
गोविन्दाङ्घ्रिसरोजध्यानसुधाजलधौतसमस्ताघो
गोविन्दं परमानन्दामृतमन्तःस्थं स तमभ्येति ॥

govindāṣṭakam etad adhīte govindārpita-cetā yo
govindācyuta mādhava viṣṇo gokula-nāyaka kṛṣṇeti
govindāṅghri-saroja-dhyāna-sudhā-jala-dhauta-samastāgho
govindaṁ paramānandāmṛtam antaḥ-sthaṁ sa tam abhyeti

Anyone who recites this *Govindāṣṭakam*, who fixes his mind on Govinda, and who sweetly chants, 'O Govinda, Acyuta, Mādhava, Viṣṇu, Gokula-nāyaka, Kṛṣṇa,' thus cleansing away all his sins with the ambrosial water of meditation on the lotus feet of Lord Govinda-such a soul will certainly attain Lord Govinda, the supreme, everlasting bliss of the heart.

Modern enlightened masters who are thought to be non-dualistic have shown pure devotion to their Iṣṭa-devatās. Nisargadhata Mahārāja performed *pūjā* daily on the orders of his master. Śrī Bhagavān Ramaṇa Maharṣi was a great devotee of Śiva; he worshipped Śiva's personification as a hill called Arunāchala. He composed a famous 108-verse devotional hymn for Lord Arunāchala Śiva in Tamil called *akṣara-mana-mālai*, written out of *mādhurya-bhāva*, meaning romantic love, which begins as follows:

அருணா அருணமணி கிரானா வலிநிகர்
தரும் அக்ஷர மனமகிழ் மாலை
தெருள்நாடியதிரு அடியர்த்தெருமரல்
தெளியபரவுதல் பொருளாக
கருணாகரமுனி ரமணாரியன்
உவகையினால் சொலியது கதியாக
அருணாச்சலமென அகமே அறிவொடும்
ஆள்வார் சிவனுலகு.. ஆள்வாரே..

tarunārunamani kiranāvalinihar, taruma ksharamana mahizhmālai
terunādiyatiru vadiyār terumaral, teliyap paravudal porulāha
karunākaramuni ramanāriyanuva, haiyinār soliyadu gatiyāha
arunāchalamena ahamēyarivodu, mazhvār śivanula hālvārē

This joyful marital garland of letters, which resembles a beam of the rays of the rising sun, was sung by the noble sage, Ramaṇa, the ocean of compassion, with the object of removing the delusion of the devotees who sought his grace. Those who look upon it as their sole refuge will realize within themselves that they are Arunāchala and will reign in the world of Śiva.

அருணாச்சல வரற்கு ஏற்ற
அக்ஷரமணமாலை சாற்றக்
கருணாகர கணபதியே
கரம் அருளிக் காப்பாயே

arunāchala vararkētra, aksharamana mālaisātra
karunākara ganapatiyē, karamarulik kāppāyē

Gracious Gaṇapati with thy (loving) hand bless me, that I may make this marital garland of letters worthy of Śrī Arunāchala, the bridegroom!

அருணாச்சலசிவ அருணாச்சலசிவ
அருணாச்சலசிவ அருணாச்சலா !

arunāchala śiva, arunāchala śiva, arunāchala śiva, arunāchala!
arunāchala śiva, arunāchala śiva, arunāchala śiva, arunāchala!

Both Ramakṛṣna Paramahaṁsa and his disciple Swami Vivekananda were great *jñanīs* and also attained the highest levels of devotion. My Paraṁ Guru, the master of my Guru Mahārāja, H.D.G. Bhagavān Avadhūta Śrī Mastarāma

Bābājī Mahārāja, composed the following devotional poem about Śrīmatī Rādhāranī in Hindi:

प्रगट भई राधिका
गंगाकी तरंग-सी
मधुरी उमंग-सी
प्रेमकी-सी व्यंजना
उदित भ ई राधिका ॥

pragaṭ bhaī rādhikā
gangākī tarang-sī
madhurī umang-sī
premkī-sī vyanjanā
udit bhaī rādhikā

Rādhikā has appeared.
She is like a wave of the Gaṅgā.
She is like an ecstasy of sweetness.
She is like an embellishment of love.
Rādhikā has manifested

प्रगट भई राधिका
कामधेनु दुग्धसी
भावमयी मुग्धसी
रासकी प्रकाशिका
उदित भई राधिका ॥

pragaṭ bhaī rādhikā

kāma-dhenu dugdhasī
bhava-mayī mugdhasī
rāsakī prakāśikā
udit bhaī rādhikā

Rādhikā has appeared.
She is a like the milk of the wish-fulfilling cow.
She is entirely divine love,
Like a tender and innocent girl.
She is the light of the *rāsa*.
Rādhikā has manifested.

प्रगट भई राधिका
विरहविलासिनि
वृंदावनवासिनि
कृष्णचंद्र चन्द्रिका
उदित भई राधिका ॥

pragaṭ bhaī rādhikā
viraha-vilāsini
vṛndāvana-vāsini
kṛṣṇa-candra candrikā
udit bhaī rādhikā

Rādhikā has appeared.
She plays love games of separation.
She dwells in Vṛndāvana.
She is the moon light,
of the moon like Kṛṣṇa.
Rādhikā has manifested.

प्रगट भई राधिका
कारुण्य लहराने
विराग बरसाने
कीरतिकी दुहिता
उदित भई राधिका ॥

pragaṭ bhaī rādhikā
kāruṇy laharāne
virāg barasāne
kīratikī duhitā
udit bhaī rādhikā

Rādhikā has appeared.
She radiates compassion.
She showers forth dispassion.
The milkmaid daughter of Kīrti,
Rādhikā has manifested.

To benefit from any yoga path, proper guidance is required. If followed properly, all paths confer considerable benefits. The contribution of bhakti yoga to the retroprogressive path is invaluable. However, it can also be dangerous and even harmful without expert advice. Improperly walked, the path of devotion can lead to religious fanaticism and stagnation on the objective plane.

Even without devotion it is possible to recognize consciousness, at least theoretically. Since what is apparent does not influence what is real, dual illusion does not affect non-dual reality. Devotion is not a requirement for realizing God, just as love is not indispensable to marry.

On marriage license applications, there is no checkbox to indicate if the couple is in love. However, a couple without love will not be able to establish a loving home. Likewise, realizing God without devotion will lack ecstasy.

Because love is an end in itself, it cannot be a means to achieve something. If you have a clear motive for loving someone, you are obviously not in love. Bhakti is not necessary to become enlightened. However, after enlightenment, apparent duality beautifies non-dual reality with devotional exchanges.

Vyāsa's dissatisfaction will help us understand this matter. He is one of the most revered figures in the *Sanātana-dharma* religion and considered to be a divine literary incarnation. He is sometimes called Veda-vyāsaḥ, or "he who compiled the Vedas." He is one of the eight immortals, or *ciranjīvin*, author of the *Vedānta Sūtra* or *Brahma-sūtra*, and composer of the *Purāṇas*. Despite his transcendental status, Vyāsa suffered from deep dissatisfaction. While he was sitting in sorrow on the banks of the Sarasvatī river, Nārada Muni appeared, who noticed his emotional state and said these words to him:

जिज्ञासितं सुसम्पन्नमपि ते महदद्भुतम् ।
कृतवान्भारतं यस्त्वं सर्वार्थपरिबृंहितम् ॥

jijñāsitaṁ susampannam
api te mahad-adbhutam
kṛtavān bhārataṁ yas tvaṁ
sarvārtha-paribṛṁhitam

Your inquiries were full and your studies were also well fulfilled, and there is no doubt that you have prepared a great and wonderful work, the *Mahābhārata*, which is full of all kinds of Vedic sequences elaborately explained.

(*Śrīmad-bhāgavatam*, 1.5.3)

जिज्ञासितमधीतं च ब्रह्म यत्तत्सनातनम् ।
तथापि शोचस्यात्मानमकृतार्थ इव प्रभो ॥

jijñāsitam adhītaṁ ca
brahma yat tat sanātanam
tathāpi śocasy ātmānam
akṛtārtha iva prabho

You have fully delineated the subject of impersonal Brahman as well as the knowledge derived therefrom. Why should you be despondent in spite of all this, thinking that you are undone, my dear prabhu?

(*Śrīmad-bhāgavatam*, 1.5.4)

Failing to understand the reason for his grief, Vyāsa asked the sage Nārada:

व्यास उवाच-
अस्त्येव मे सर्वमिदं त्वयोक्तं
तथापि नात्मा परितुष्यते मे ।
तन्मूलमव्यक्तमगाधबोधं
पृच्छामहे त्वात्मभवात्मभूतम् ॥

vyāsa uvāca
asty eva me sarvam idaṁ tvayoktaṁ
tathāpi nātmā parituṣyate me
tan-mūlam avyaktam agādha-bodhaṁ
pṛcchāmahe tvātma-bhavātma-bhūtam

Śrī Vyāsadeva said: "All you have said about me is perfectly correct. Despite all this, I am not pacified. I therefore question you about the root cause of my dissatisfaction, for you are a man of unlimited knowledge due to your being the offspring of one [Brahmā] who is self-born [without mundane father and mother]."

(*Śrīmad-bhāgavatam*, 1.5.5)

Vyāsa was fully aware of the excellent virtues that Nārada mentioned. However, something was missing: poetry, dance, madness, fire, and ecstasy. Nārada Muni's reply was blunt and direct: however transcendental your position may be, you have forgotten love. Despite your sainthood and high status, you have forgotten bhakti.

यथा धर्मादयश्चार्था मुनिवर्यानुकीर्तिताः ।
न तथा वासुदेवस्य महिमा ह्यनुवर्णितः ॥

yathā dharmādayaś cārthā
muni-varyānukīrtitāḥ
na tathā vāsudevasya
mahimā hy anuvarṇitaḥ

Although, great sage, you have very broadly described the four principles beginning with religious performances, you have not described the glories of the Supreme Personality, Vāsudeva.

(*Śrīmad-bhāgavatam*, 1.5.9)

न यद्वचश्चित्रपदं हरेर्यशो
जगत्पवित्रं प्रगृणीत कर्हिचित् ।
तद्वायसं तीर्थमुशन्ति मानसा
न यत्र हंसा निरमन्त्युशिक्क्षयाः ॥

na yad vacaś citra-padaṁ harer yaśo
jagat-pavitraṁ pragṛṇīta karhicit
tad vāyasaṁ tīrtham uśanti mānasā
na yatra haṁsā niramanty uśik-kṣayāḥ

Those words which do not describe the glories of the Lord, who alone can sanctify the atmosphere of the whole universe, are considered by saintly persons to be like unto a place of pilgrimage for crows. Since the all-perfect persons are inhabitants of the transcendental abode, they do not derive any pleasure there.

(*Śrīmad-bhāgavatam*, 1.5.10)

तद्वाग्विसर्गो जनताघविप्लवो
यस्मिन्प्रतिश्लोकमबद्धवत्यपि ।
नामान्यनन्तस्य यशोऽङ्कितानि यत्
शृण्वन्ति गायन्ति गृणन्ति साधवः ॥

tad-vāg-visargo janatāgha-viplavo
yasmin prati-ślokam abaddhavaty api
nāmāny anantasya yaśo 'ṅkitāni yat
śṛṇvanti gāyanti gṛṇanti sādhavaḥ

> On the other hand, that literature which is full of descriptions of the transcendental glories of the name, fame, forms, pastimes, etc., of the unlimited Supreme Lord is a different creation, full of transcendental words directed toward bringing about a revolution in the impious lives of this world's misdirected civilization. Such transcendental literatures, even though imperfectly composed, are heard, sung, and accepted by purified men who are thoroughly honest.
>
> (*Śrīmad-bhāgavatam*, 1.5.11)

Nārada's advice to Vyāsa was to recall Kṛṣṇa's divine pastimes and describe them for the benefit of the public. This is how the *Bhāgavata Purāṇa* or *Śrīmad-bhāgavatam* was born.

Śrī Ramākṛṣṇa Paramahaṁsa, a great master and devotee of Mother Kālī, used to say in describing the personal form of higher consciousness, "I want to taste sugar, not become sugar." Although we are essentially sweetness itself, we opt for the enjoyment of it through apparent contraction and identification.

In egoic devotion, there is a separate "I" that feels.

However, genuine bhakti is an invitation to disappear into the beloved. The experience of a feeling "I" that experiences emotions for God or the guru may just be egoic sentimentality. This type of bhakti is dangerous because we can stagnate in egoic emotions. A major problem is that intellectual ignorance is more noticeable than emotional ignorance. It is easier to identify an incorrect thought than an incorrect emotion. Egoic religious emotions arise from what is apparent, relative, dual, private, and personal, while Advaitic bhakti is an expression of non-duality. Rather than emotion, it is devotion.

In the commentary on mantra 17, we mentioned that according to Aristotle, God is only *nóesis noéseos,* or "a thought that thinks itself." Such thinking is not a mental activity; God thinks about himself like a thought that thinks itself. This is a fixed thought because it lacks the process of transformation of the potency into act. God is only actualization, or *energeia* (ἐνέργεια). We can apply Aristotle's metaphysics, but replace *thought* with *love,* since "God is love" (1 John, 4:8). The One without a second can only love itself. Since Kṛṣṇa is the only reality that exists, he can only love himself. Therefore, Kṛṣṇa would not only be love, but a love that loves himself. By loving himself, he emerges as subjective diversity: simultaneously the one who loves and the one who is loved. The worshipper is the worshipped. Rādhā loves Kṛṣṇa.

রাধাকৃষ্ণ এক আত্মা, দুই দেহ ধরি' ।
অন্যোন্যে বিলসে রস আস্বাদন করি' ॥

rādhā-kṛṣṇa eka ātmā, dui deha dhari'
anyonye vilase rasa āsvādana kari'

Rādhā and Kṛṣṇa are one and the same, but they have assumed two bodies. Thus, they enjoy each other, tasting the mellows of love.
(*Śrī Caitanya-caritāmṛta*, "*Ādi-līlā*," 4.56)

সেই প্রেমার শ্রীরাধিকা পরম 'আশ্রয়' ।
সেই প্রেমার আমি হই কেবল 'বিষয়' ॥

sei premāra śrī-rādhikā parama 'āśraya'
sei premāra āmi ha-i kevala 'viṣaya'

Śrī Rādhikā is the highest abode of that love, and I am its only object.
(*Śrī Caitanya-caritāmṛta*, "*Ādi-līlā*," 4.132)

বিষয়জাতীয় সুখ আমার আস্বাদ ।
আমা হৈতে কোটিগুণ আশ্রয়ের আহ্লাদ ॥

viṣaya-jātīya sukha āmāra āsvāda
āmā haite koṭi-guṇa āśrayera āhlāda

I taste the bliss to which the object of love is entitled. But the pleasure of Rādhā, the abode of

that love, is ten million times greater.
(*Śrī Caitanya-caritāmṛta*, "*Ādi-līlā*," 4.133)

কভু যদি এই প্রেমার হইয়ে আশ্রয় ।
তবে এই প্রেমানন্দের অনুভব হয় ॥

kabhu yadi ei premāra ha-iye āśraya
tabe ei premānandera anubhava haya

If sometimes I can be the abode of that love, only then may I taste its joy.
(*Śrī Caitanya-caritāmṛta*, "*Ādi-līlā*," 4.135)

এত চিন্তি' রহে কৃষ্ণ পরমকৌতুকী ।
হৃদয়ে বাড়য়ে প্রেম-লোভ ধক্‌ধকি ॥

eta cinti' rahe kṛṣṇa parama-kautukī
hṛdaye bāḍaye prema-lobha dhakdhaki

Thinking in this way, Lord Kṛṣṇa was curious to taste that love. His eager desire for that love increasingly blazed in his heart.
(*Śrī Caitanya-caritāmṛta*, "*Ādi-līlā*," 4.136)

All great realized masters do not love God but disappear in their beloved. Retroprogressive bhakti, or true devotion, unlike religious sentimentalism, emanates from the innermost non-duality. The very subjective duality of worshipper-worshipped arises and dissolves in love.

प्रायेण मुनयो राजन्निवृत्ता विधिषेधतः ।
नैर्गुण्यस्था रमन्ते स्म गुणानुकथने हरेः ॥

prāyeṇa munayo rājan
nivṛttā vidhi-ṣedhataḥ
nairguṇya-sthā ramante sma
guṇānukathane hareḥ

O King Parīkṣit, mainly the topmost transcendentalists, who are above the regulative principles and restrictions, take pleasure in describing the glories of the Lord.

(*Śrīmad-bhāgavatam*, 2.1.7)

Saint Thomas Aquinas writes:

Therefore, when an entity in which a given good exists is more noble than the soul itself, in which the nature as understood exists, then the will is higher than the intellect in relation to such an entity. But when the entity in which a given good exists is inferior to the soul, then the intellect is higher than the will in relation to such an entity. Hence, the love of God is better than the cognition of God, whereas, conversely, the cognition of corporeal things is better than the love of corporeal things. Still, absolutely speaking, the intellect is more noble than the will.

(*Summa Theologiae*, I, q. 82, a. 3.)

"Guide us to wealth..."

This last verse of the *Īśāvāsya Upanishad* begins by referring to the same sacrificial fire used for cremation. The sage begs Agni, who guides souls after death, to lead him on the right path to wealth. Of course, the yogi is not asking to be guided so he can acquire jewels or diamonds. Once humans obtain material wealth, they understand the price of the success they longed for. The Greek philosopher Epicurus of Samos said: "If you wish to be rich, do not strive to increase your possessions, but to decrease your greed."

Many strive to hoard wealth throughout their lives and hope to finally rest the day they obtain it. Their lives are dominated by nervousness, restlessness, worry, and anxiety. After a life of anguish, tension becomes second nature. When they grow old, they might have achieved wealth, but they are unable to relax and enjoy the peace and quiet they yearned for. By neglecting non-monetary aspects of life due to a lack of time, they have undermined their sensitivity. Since they have devoted their lives to making money, they have forgotten to contemplate the stars, walk along the seashore, and sit in the forest to enjoy the sound of the breeze in the trees, because none of this earns dollars, rupees, or pesos. Since they have taken every opportunity to make money, they have not prioritized meeting people, making real friends, and enjoying poetry, painting, dance, and music. They have opted to postpone all that until they have enough wealth to be able to relax and sit back and enjoy those aspects of life. Only then do they realize that, although they have obtained what they desired, they have actually lost something much more essential.

The pursuit of wealth completely transmutes human beings. Once people obtain the wealth they desire, they are transformed into beings with no sensitivity. They are unable to vibrate with the stars, the moon, and the sea. After years of chasing money, they lose the sensibility to enjoy music, comprehend poetry, and they become clumsy dancers. In reality, they have been transformed into beings whose only strength is obtaining something that does not bring joy. To earn a lot of money, they were forced to ignore their receptivity and after having hoarded millions, they see that their heart has atrophied. They possess a lot, but they have lost their delicacy of spirit and innate capacity for enjoyment.

In order to cultivate a delicate sensitivity that is capable of being touched by a sunset or a seagull in the sky, we need free time. Those who aspire to wealth often lack the time to cultivate their sensitivity. One problem for celebrities, famous singers, and successful soccer players is that they have a lot of money but not enough time to enjoy it. They are too busy touring or training. Only then do they realize that economic wealth brings great poverty. They are so poor that they have nothing but money. They finally recognize that what is really valuable in this life has no price. As Canadian actor James Eugene Carrey said: "I think everybody should get rich and famous and do everything they ever dreamed of so they can see that it's not the answer."

Life itself is priceless. And if we waste life running after wealth, we are accepting a very bad deal. To obtain money, what we invest is our very life. Our salary is earned with hours, weeks, months, and years of our lives. The problem is that life slips away and it is impossible to buy back even one second. José Luis López Aranguren was one of the most influential Spanish philosophers and essayists of the twentieth century. He said: "We seek happiness in external goods, in riches, and consumerism is the current form of the ultimate good. But the image of the satisfied consumer is illusory: consumers are never satisfied; they are insatiable and, therefore, unhappy. We can seek happiness in success, fame, and honors. But isn't all that nothing but vanity, that is, nothing or almost nothing?"

Obviously, I do not condemn honest labor and wealth, nor do I advise renouncing possessions. I am only saying that it is essential to cultivate the art of inner wealth. And this art begins by finding the meaning of life and being present in each and every one of our actions.

The pursuit of wealth comes from the drive to transcend our limits. When we look at ourselves in the mirror, we see a form limited by space and time. Yet something within us whispers softly in our ear that we are something more. This dissatisfaction stems from a deep sense of limitation. We desire a larger car, a bigger house, a higher bank balance, and more and more, *ad infinitum*. The more we get, the more we want. When we identify with the gross body, we yearn for what gives us the most sensory pleasure. When we identify with the mind and intellect, we seek to accumulate knowledge. When we identify with our feelings, we want romance and all kinds of emotional experiences. Only by glimpsing the soul do our aspirations and ambitions focus on the spirit. The pursuit of certain kinds of possessions—physical, intellectual, psychological, emotional, and spiritual—largely depends on our evolutionary level, and thus, on our level of *viveka*, or "power of discrimination." Searching transforms seekers, whether or not they find what they are looking for. If you seek the Truth, you will be completely transformed, even if you do not find it. If you seek God, the search will totally change your life, even if you do not reach self-realization.

"... on the right path."

Society has implanted in us the idea that we must strive to be someone in life and improve, progress, advance, and succeed, even at the cost of stepping over others. This attitude has become part of our nature, poisoning our being, and giving us no respite.

All goals are illusory ideas that push us to abandon the present to live in the future. The hope of arriving at a safe harbor keeps us focused on the future, stripping value from the present. Our attention is focused on illusory goals, and we ignore the reality of the here and now.

The here loses its magic, the now becomes ordinary, and life loses its charm. Goals reside in our imagination; they are only a projection of our past. However, these illusory goals become more important than the present moment, which is real. When our life is motivated by a dream, disappointment awaits us at the end of the road. A fantasy cannot be achieved. No matter how hard we try, the fantasy will always be just that: an illusion. We will waste our real life trying to realize a dream in a tomorrow that will never come.

The path I am proposing is aimless. There is no place to arrive and there is no one who will arrive. The retroprogressive path is a path without a goal. We call it a *path* because it has a direction, even though it lacks a destination. Neither Truth, nor God, nor enlightenment are goals: they are already in us, here and in the present moment. The problem is that most of us are not present and, therefore, we do not find Truth. Enlightenment awaits us here and now, but we are lost in the nostalgia of the past and in the expectations of a distant future.

The Hebrew revelation has the beautiful term *teshuvah*, or "to return." One who follows the spiritual path is not going toward a goal in the future but going back. I propose the retroprogressive path, which is a return to our eternal home. It is a return to where we really are, to the here and now.

בָּרוּךְ אַתָּה ה' אֱלֹקֵינוּ מֶלֶךְ הָעוֹלָם, שֶׁהֶחֱיָנוּ וְקִיְּמָנוּ וְהִגִּיעָנוּ לַזְּמַן הַזֶּה.

> *baruch atah, Hashem Elokeinu, Melech haolam, she'hecheyanu, ve'kiymanu, ve'higianu lazman hazeh.*
>
> Blessed are You, God our Lord, sovereign of all, who has kept us alive, sustained us, and brought us to this time.

On the spiritual path, there is no goal, because we already are what we aspire to be. We have never ceased to be what we wish to be, not even for a moment. We have always been reality or the Self. Any focus on external goals will distract us from the reality of the present and life. My message is an invitation to strip ourselves of any purpose. What I suggest is dispensing with goals and placing ourselves in this very moment, as it is. There is no goal, but there is direction. And the direction is not north or south, east or west, but toward what enriches us and shows us our inner treasure. In reality, the only direction is inward.

There is a "right" or "adequate" path to wealth. Often, the problem is not what we want, but the means to attain it. Wanting to watch television is not wrong, but stealing a television is wrong. Desiring money is acceptable; scamming others is not. Wanting to have sex is not a sin, but cheating, abusing, and raping is. If we wish to transcend our limitations and realize our divine nature, there is a proper path. The expression "right path" may suggest that Truth does not lie in the present, but somewhere in the future. But Truth is not an object and knowing it does not mean possessing it. Truth is a mystery to be realized, discovered, and unveiled.

The wrong path offers a static goal and, consequently, requires discipline and greed as means to achieve the goal. These qualities rob us of our freedom and condition our lives. Seeing Truth as a distant goal, accessible only through practice, leads to imitation and dependence on someone to guide us. This imitation is disguised as inquiry.

The search for Truth as a static goal is not the search for God but for security. The wrong path is to pursue security. To attain it, the mind seeks a methodology and a set of techniques to be followed to the letter, which completely conditions the mind through control and repression. But Truth is not the result or product of a specific type of conditioning. The right path is constant realization, free from a static goal. The right path invites us on the adventure of revealing our inner treasure and makes us less false and more authentic with every step.

"O, knower of our activities!"

The Vedantic sage addresses consciousness as the "knower of our activities." Fascinated by objective reality, we forget our authentic nature. We think we are the doers of what happens to us. The evolutionary process leading to the realization of ultimate reality is intimately connected to self-observation. Along with observation, we overcome the illusion that we are the doer and adopt a new position as the witness of our activities and experiences. Retroprogressive wisdom does not change experiences, but our approach to them. By observing, we move from being based purely in ego to the dimension of consciousness.

The ego, as the supposed doer, interprets and judges. It escapes uncomfortable experiences and strives for pleasurable ones. The limited "I" does not observe; it interprets what appears on its horizon based on previous experiences and appropriates what happens. While consciousness observes, the separate "I" lives immersed in identification with acquired beliefs and traditions, beginning early in childhood. Its reactions reproduce old stories, scenarios, and dramas that lead it to play out old and painful roles. It reenacts stories full of fear, pain, loneliness, abandonment, disappointments, and abuse. The identification with these old scripts is so deep that it seems impossible to overcome it. The egoic phenomenon is an almost hypnotic state. In it, there is a firm conviction that we are these imaginary roles, but they mask our true identity. The mask is our personality. The ego's old dramas captivate us and hold us in a dream that is very difficult to wake up from. The end of the dream is waking up to the now, to the present, and to the reality of what is, as it is.

Basing ourselves on a synthesis of Salvador Pániker, Martin Heidegger, and Jean Paul Gustave Ricoeur, we could say that our attraction to the present comes from our attempts to escape pain. Our vague suspicion that time does not exist makes us think that if we mentally place ourselves in the present, the anguish of past events will disappear. When we listen to the ancestral guidance of the great masters, who advise living in the present, we try to place our minds in the now, which is a false strategy. However, some false strategies have seeds of truth: hiding the unpleasant side of things is a caricatured way of foreseeing that yesterday and tomorrow do not exist. By "situating ourselves in the now," I am not referring to Horace's *carpe diem*, or "seize the day" (*Odes*, 11.8), which some people use incorrectly to justify reckless behavior.

The mind can think about the present, but it cannot really situate itself in the now. Thought can imagine the present, but not establish itself in it. The human being, as an egoic phenomenon, is a tension between yesterday and tomorrow, between what has been and what will be. Everything negative resides in memory and imagination: painful memories and dreaded outcomes. Thus, Heidegger conceptualizes being as "a future which becomes present in the process of having been." This includes past, present, and future. This idea has such a profound impact on us because it is so similar to the unutterable sacred term for divinity in the Sinaitic revelation, YHWH (ה-ו-ה-י), which encompasses all that was, is, and will be.

Heidegger arrives at this interesting concept from Edmund Husserl's *On the Phenomenology of the Consciousness of Internal Time*. The key terms are *proto-impression, retention,* and *protention*. The mind has three functions that perceive present, past, and future.

1. *Proto-impression* is when the mind has the intention to assimilate new material in the present moment.
2. *Retention* is when the mind is directed at what was already received, maintaining a present directed toward the past.
3. *Protention* is the mind directed to the future.

Human beings emerge out of the tension between these three functions. The egoic phenomenon is a tension between the present, memory, and expectations. The separate "I" is a tension between what is, what was, and what will be, that is, between what is experienced, what was experienced, and what is expected from future experiences.

In philosophical terms, the unconscious symbolizes concealing all that is negative. We usually show what we think is positive, while we tend to hide what we see as negative, harmful, detrimental, or damaging. In a fundamental phenomenological and hermeneutical analysis, we see how guilt, pain, and resentment chain us to the past. Guilt comes from the hurt we have caused. We store it in the unconscious because we refuse to recognize the pain we have caused. Living with guilty feelings is a constant ordeal, accompanied by unpleasant emotions such as anguish, frustration, sadness, and remorse. Pain comes from injuries that we have endured. Lastly, resentment is accumulated hatred for not having avenged offenses we have suffered, according to Max Scheler.

> When they kept on questioning him, he straightened up and said to them, "Let any one of you who is without sin be the first to throw a stone at her."
>
> (New Testament, John, 8:7)

Edmund Husserl uses the term retention for guilt, pain, and resentment because they keep us tied to the past. Freeing ourselves from them is only possible by transcending the unconscious and going beyond the mind.

On the other hand, anguish, fear, and despair chain us to the future.

Anguish is the threat of the nothingness that awaits us when we die. Phenomenologically, death for human beings is the threat of being nullified forever. With every second of life, we are closer to death or eternal "nullification." All minds are overwhelmed with anguish over the possibility of disappearing forever.

Fear is born out of concern for all that is to come. Human beings feel fragile in the face of life's uncertainty. We are afraid of what may happen. Fear appears when we think of possible suffering, illness, or pain. While fear is over everything, anguish is over nothing. Since it is nothingness, death causes anguish, not fear. Fear is animalistic and anguish is human. Fear is instinctive and anguish is intellectual.

Finally, despair binds us to the future. The source of our despair is knowing that we may do harm. I do not intend to deny that the structure of the unconscious has to do with language, but it is also a force that pushes us to make irrational choices. The unconscious is the irresistible power of repeating both healthy and unhealthy habits. Out of this fear, Arjuna asks Kṛṣṇa:

> अर्जुन उवाच-
> अथ केन प्रयुक्तोऽयं पापं चरति पूरुषः ।
> अनिच्छन्नपि वार्ष्णेय बलादिव नियोजितः ॥

> *arjuna uvāca*
> *atha kena prayukto 'yaṁ*
> *pāpaṁ carati pūruṣaḥ*
> *anicchann api vārṣṇeya*
> *balād iva niyojitaḥ*

> Arjuna said: "O descendant of Vṛṣṇi, what impels us to sinful acts, even unwillingly, as if obliged by some force?"
>
> (Bhagavad Gita, 3.36)

"Liberate us from the attraction to sin."

In Hebrew, the original language of the Bible, the word for sin is *chet*, which means "error or mistake," in the sense of not reaching a goal, objective, or certain target. This denotes an attitude rather than a sin. It would be imprudent to condemn someone to hell just because of a mistake. Sins are not about what we have done, but our level of consciousness. Thus, the source of all sin is unconsciousness, just as the source of all virtue is consciousness. Even if we do good deeds, they will not be virtuous if they come from our illusion. Freeing ourselves from the attraction to sin is only possible when we develop consciousness. Then, we will not commit sins or makes mistakes. Consciousness comes with the clarity required to avoid any harm to others. Sinners are sleepwalkers who, although they seem awake, act based on their dreams. Clearly, they will bump into chairs and crash into walls and people. Awakening is the only way to free ourselves from sin. A being of consciousness is a light to the world, a light to the nations.

The only way to awaken and transcend the mental plane is attentive observation. Meditation is another name for observation. Many people talk about meditation as a science, technique, or method. However, meditation is an art, game, or occupation that we do without expecting a reward. It is an activity that we perform motivated by the pleasure of the work itself, without expecting any result from our action. I am thinking of activities like dancing, singing, writing, painting, and playing sports like golf or tennis. Meditation is the only cognitive activity that is totally independent of the mind. It is not another mental activity such as reflecting, thinking, imagining, or speculating. To meditate is to observe and know our activities in any field. Observation begins with the disidentification of the mind and adopting the position of a witness. Only observation allows us to create a distance and, therefore, a disidentification from what is observed.

To meditate is to watch, observe, and know our activities and experiences at all levels: physical, mental, emotional, and energetic. The most immediate level of identification is the physical one. Hatha yoga is observing the body, gradually moving toward disidentification. Observing our arms, legs, and back as they touch the mat. Observing the breath in the nostrils and noticing that the air we inhale is cooler than the air we exhale. Observing our breathing without intervening or trying to control it.

On the mental level, we observe our mind and its activity without analyzing it. We allow ideas, emotions, thoughts, feelings, and all kinds of sensations to parade at their own pace without interpreting them. We only observe without defining, judging, analyzing, controlling, or elucidating what we observe. Meditation consists of attentive observation with absolute neutrality. Observation empties the mind and, at the same time, creates a state of alertness, of keen attention. We then experience a mental emptiness along with the clarity of awakening. Consequently, mental activity decreases as attention increases. At a certain point, we will be able to observe ourselves, that is to say, to see our small "I" as a simple idea, thought, or emotion. We will then cease to be a witness, or someone who observes, and awaken to our reality as pure observation. We will be participants in the realization that observation is consciousness. We will awaken to our reality, no longer as the doer, and not even as the observer, but as observation itself.

Sanskrit Pronunciation Guide

The Sanskrit Alphabet

Vowels

अ *a* आ *ā* इ *i* ई *ī* उ *u* ऊ *ū*
ऋ *ṛ* ॠ *ṝ* ऌ *ḷ* ए *e* ऐ *ai* ओ *o* औ *au* अं *aṁ* अः *aḥ*

Consonants

Gutturals	क *ka*	ख *kha*	ग *ga*	घ *gha*	ङ ṅa
Palatals	च *ca*	छ *cha*	ज *ja*	झ *jha*	ञ ña
Cerebrals	ट *ṭa*	ठ *ṭha*	ड *ḍa*	ढ *ḍha*	ण ṇa
Dentals	त *ta*	थ *tha*	द *da*	ध *dha*	न na
Labials	प *pa*	फ *pha*	ब *ba*	भ *bha*	म ma
Semivowels	य *ya*	र *ra*	ल *la*	व *va*	
Sibilants	श *śa*	ष *ṣa*	स *sa*		
Aspirates	ह *ha*				

Pronunciation

Vowels

Sanskrit letter	Transliteration	Sounds like
अ	*a*	but
आ	*ā*	father
इ	*i*	fit, if, lily
ई	*ī*	fee, police
उ	*u*	put
ऊ	*ū*	boot, rule, rude
ऋ	*ṛ*	(between ri and ru, as in the name Krishna)
ॠ	*ṝ*	(between ri and ru) crucial
ऌ	*ḷ*	(similar to lr)
ए	*e*	made
ऐ	*ai*	bite, aisle
ओ	*o*	oh
औ	*au*	found, house

Consonants

Gutturals

(back of the throat)

Sanskrit letter	Transliteration	Sounds like
क	*ka*	kill, seek, kite
ख	*kha*	Eckhart
ग	*ga*	get, dog, give
घ	*gha*	log-hut
ङ	*ṅa*	sing, king, sink

Palatals

(tip of the tongue touches the roof of the mouth)

Sanskrit letter	Transliteration	Sounds like
च	*ca*	chicken
छ	*cha*	catch him
ज	*ja*	joy, jump
झ	*jha*	hedgehog
ञ	*ña*	canyon

Cerebrals

(tip of the tongue against the front part of the roof of the mouth)

Sanskrit letter	Transliteration	Sounds like
ट	*ṭa*	true, tub
ठ	*ṭha*	anthill
ड	*ḍa*	dove, drum, doctor
ढ	*ḍha*	red-hot
ण	*ṇa*	under

Dentals

(tip of the tongue against the teeth)

Sanskrit letter	Transliteration	Sounds like
त	*ta*	(between t and th) water
थ	*tha*	lighthearted
द	*da*	(between d and th) dice, then
ध	*dha*	adhere
न	*na*	not, nut

Labials

(lips together, the tongue is not used)

Sanskrit letter	Transliteration	Sounds like
प	*pa*	pine, put, sip
फ	*pha*	uphill
ब	*ba*	bird, bear, rub
भ	*bha*	abhor
म	*ma*	mother, map

Semivowels

Sanskrit letter	Transliteration	Sounds like
य	*ya*	yet, loyal, yes
र	*ra*	red, year
ल	*la*	lull, lead
व	*va*	(between v and w)
		ivy, vine

Sibilants

Sanskrit letter	Transliteration	Sounds like
श	*śa*	sure
ष	*ṣa*	shrink, bush, show
स	*sa*	saint, sin, hiss

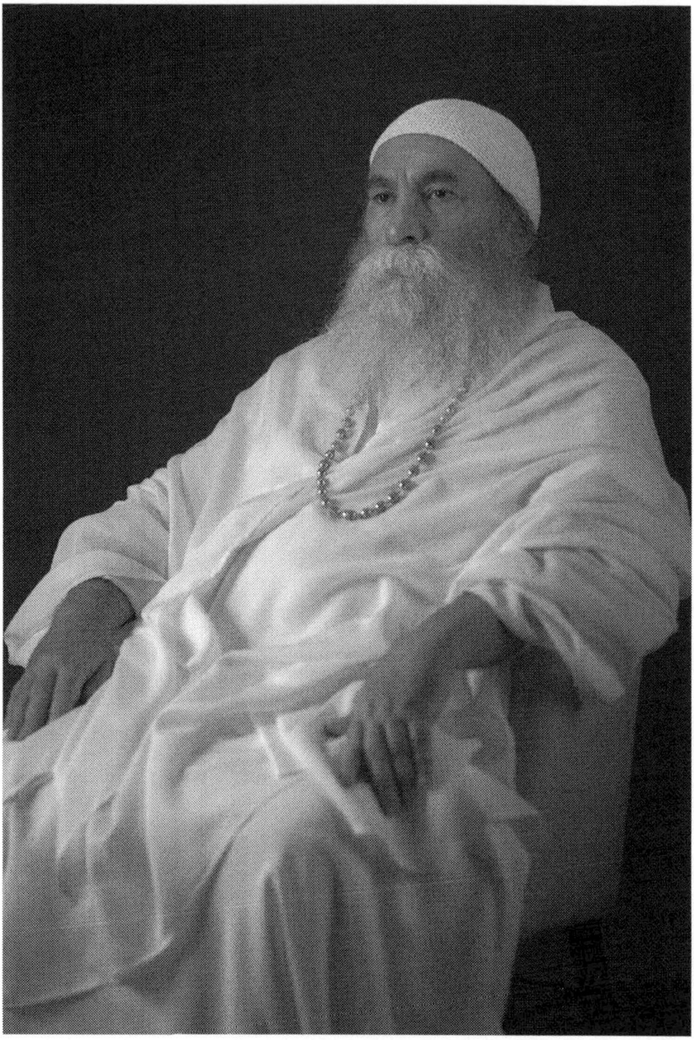

Prabhuji

S.S. Avadhūta Śrī Bhaktivedānta Yogācārya
Ramakrishnananda Bābājī Mahārāja

Biography

Prabhuji is a writer, painter, Krishnaite devotee (*Kṛṣṇa-bhakta*), *avadhūta* mystic, the creator of Retroprogressive Yoga, and a realized spiritual master. In 2011, he chose to retire from society and lead the life of a hermit. Since then, his days have been spent in solitude, praying, writing, painting, and meditating in silence and contemplation.

Prabhuji is the sole disciple of H.D.G. Avadhūta Śrī Brahmānanda Bābājī Mahārāja, who in turn is one of the closest and most intimate disciples of H.D.G. Avadhūta Śrī Mastarāma Bābājī Mahārāja.

Prabhuji was appointed as the successor of the lineage by his master, who conferred upon him the responsibility of continuing the line of disciplic succession of *avadhūtas*, or the sacred *paramparā*, officially appointing him as guru and ordering him to serve as Ācārya successor under the name H.H. Avadhūta Śrī Bhaktivedānta Yogācārya Ramakrishnananda Bābājī Mahārāja.

Prabhuji's Hinduism is so broad, universal, and pluralistic that at times, while living up to his title of *avadhūta*, his lively and fresh teachings transcend the boundaries of all philosophies and religions, even his own. His teachings promote critical thinking and lead us to question statements that are usually accepted as true. They do not defend absolute truths but invite us to evaluate and question our own convictions. The essence of his syncretic vision, Retroprogressive Yoga, is self-awareness and the recognition of consciousness. For him, awakening at the level of consciousness, or the transcendence of the egoic phenomenon, is the next step in humanity's evolution.

Prabhuji was born on March 21, 1958, in Santiago, the capital of the Republic of Chile. When he was eight years old, he had a mystical experience that motivated his search for the Truth, or the Ultimate Reality. This transformed his life into an authentic inner and outer pilgrimage. He has completely devoted his life to deepening the early transformative experience that marked the beginning of his process of retroevolution. He has dedicated more than fifty years to the exploration and practice of different religions, philosophies, paths of liberation, and spiritual disciplines. He has absorbed the teachings of great yogis, pastors, rabbis, monks, gurus, philosophers, sages, and saints whom he personally visited during years of searching. He has lived in many places and traveled the world thirsting for Truth.

From an early age, Prabhuji noticed that the educational system prevented him from devoting himself to what was really important: learning about himself. Despite his parents' insistence, he stopped attending conventional school at the age of 11 and engaged in autodidactic formation. Over time, he would become a serious critic of the current educational system.

Prabhuji is a recognized authority on Eastern wisdom. He is known for his erudition in the *Vaidika* and *Tāntrika* aspects of Hinduism and all branches of yoga (*jñāna, karma*, *bhakti*, *haṭha*, *rāja*, *kuṇḍalinī*, tantra, mantra, and others). He has an inclusive attitude toward all religions and is intimately familiar with Judaism, Christianity, Buddhism, Sufism, Taoism, Sikhism, Jainism, Shintoism, Bahaism, and the Mapuche religion, among others. He learned about the Druze religion directly from Salach Abbas and Kamil Shchadi.

His curiosity for Western thought led him to venture into the field of philosophy. He had the privilege of studying intensively for several years with his uncle Jorge Balazs, philosopher, researcher, writer, and author of *The Golden Deer*. He studied privately with Dr. Jonathan Ramos, a renowned philosopher, historian, and university professor graduated from the Catholic University of Salta, Argentina. He also studied intensively with Dr. Alejandro Cavallazzi Sánchez, who holds an undergraduate degree in philosophy from the Universidad Panamericana, a master's degree in philosophy from the Universidad Iberoamericana, and a doctorate in philosophy from the Universidad Nacional Autónoma de México (UNAM).

Prabhuji holds a doctorate in Vaishnava philosophy from the respected Jiva Institute in Vrindavan, India, and a doctorate in yogic philosophy from the Yoga Samskrutum University.

His profound studies, his masters' blessings, his research into the sacred scriptures, and his vast teaching experience have earned him international recognition in the field of religion and spirituality.

His spiritual search led him to study with masters of diverse traditions and travel far from his native Chile to places as distant as Israel, India, and the USA. Prabhuji studied Hebrew and Sanskrit to deepen his understanding of the holy scriptures. He also studied Pali at the Oxford Centre for Buddhist Studies. Furthermore, he learned ancient Latin and Greek from Javier Álvarez, who holds a degree in Classical Philology from Sevilla University.

His father, Yosef Har-Zion ZT"L, grew up under strict discipline because he was the son of a senior police sergeant. As a reaction to this upbringing, Yosef decided to raise his own children with complete freedom and unconditional love. Prabhuji grew up without any pressure. During his early years, his father showed his son the same love regardless of his successes or failures at school. When Prabhuji decided to drop out of school in the seventh grade to devote himself to his inner quest, his family accepted his decision with deep respect. From the time his son was ten years old, Yosef talked to him about Hebrew spirituality and Western philosophy. They engaged in conversations about philosophy and religion for days on end and late into the night. Yosef supported him in whatever he wanted to do in his life and his search for Truth. Prabhuji was the authentic project of freedom and unconditional love of his father.

At an early age and on his own initiative, Prabhuji began to practice karate and study philosophy and religion. During his adolescence, no one interfered with his decisions. At the age of 15, he established a deep, intimate, and long friendship with the famous Uruguayan writer and poet Blanca Luz Brum, who was his neighbor on Merced Street in Santiago de Chile. He traveled throughout Chile in search of wise and interesting people to learn from. In southern Chile, he met machis who taught him about the rich Mapuche spirituality and shamanism.

In Chile in 1976, Prabhuji met H.D.G Bhaktikavi Atulānanda Ācārya Swami, disciple of A.C. Bhaktivedanta Swami Prabhupāda, with whom he began the initial stage of his retroprogressive process. In those days, Atulānanda Swami was a young *brahmacārī* who held the position of president of the ISKCON temple at Eyzaguirre 2404, Puente Alto, Santiago, Chile. Years later, he gave Prabhuji first initiation and Brahminical initiation. Eventually, he initiated Prabhuji into the sacred order of renunciation called *sannyāsa* within the Brahma Gauḍīya Saṁpradāya line of disciplic succession. H.D.G Bhaktikavi Atulānanda Ācārya connected him to the devotion to Kṛṣṇa. He imparted to him the wisdom of bhakti yoga and instructed him in the practice of *māhā-mantra* and the study of the holy scriptures.

Prabhuji wanted to confirm his *sannyāsa* initiation in an Advaita Vedanta lineage. His *sannyāsa-dīkṣā* was confirmed by H.H. Swami Jyotirmayānanda Sarasvatī, founder of the Yoga Research Foundation and disciple of H.H. Swami Śivānanda Sarasvatī of Rishikesh.

In 1984, he learned and began to practice Maharishi Mahesh Yogi's Transcendental Meditation technique. In 1988, he took the *kriyā-yoga* course on Paramahaṁsa Yogananda. After two years, he was officially initiated into the technique of *kriyā-yoga* by the Self-Realization Fellowship.

In 1996, Prabhuji met his guru, H.D.G. Avadhūta Śrī Brahmānanda Bābājī Mahārāja, in Rishikesh, India. Guru Mahārāja, as Prabhuji called him, revealed that his own master, H.D.G. Avadhūta Śrī Mastarāma Bābājī Mahārāja, had told him years before he died that a person would come from the West and request to be his disciple. He commanded him to accept only that particular seeker. When he asked how he would identify this person, Mastarāma Bābājī replied, "You will recognize him by his eyes. You must accept him because he will be the continuation of the lineage."

From the first moment Guru Mahārāja saw Prabhuji, he recognized him and officially initiated him into the *māhā-mantra* in Rishikesh, India. The initiation he received marked the end of a quest that began with his mystical experience at the age of eight. It also marked the beginning of the most intense and mature stage of Prabhuji's retroprogressive process. Under the guidance of Guru Mahārāja, he studied Advaita Vedanta and deepened his meditation.

The enlightened *bābājī* guided Prabhuji on his first

steps toward the sacred level of *avadhūta*. In March 2011, H.D.G. Avadhūta Śrī Brahmānanda Bābājī Mahārāja ordered Prabhuji, on behalf of his own master, to accept the responsibility of continuing the line of disciplic succession of *avadhūtas*. With this title, Prabhuji is the official representative of the line of this disciplic succession for the present generation.

Besides his *dikṣā-guru*, Prabhuji studied with important spiritual and religious personalities, such as H.H. Swami Dayananda Sarasvatī, H.H. Swami Viṣṇu Devānanda Sarasvatī, H.H. Swami Jyotirmayānanda Sarasvatī, H.H. Swami Pratyagbodhānanda, H.H. Swami Swahananda of the Ramakrishna Mission, and H.H. Swami Viditātmānanda of the Arsha Vidya Gurukulam. The wisdom of tantra was awakened in Prabhuji by H.G. Mātājī Rīnā Śarmā in India.

In Vrindavan, he did in-depth studies on the bhakti yoga path with H.H. Narahari Dāsa Bābājī Mahārāja, disciple of H.H. Nityananda Dāsa Bābājī Mahārāja of Vraja.

He also studied bhakti yoga with various disciples of His Divine Grace A.C. Bhaktivedānta Swami Prabhupāda: H.H. Kapīndra Swami, H.H. Paramadvaiti Mahārāja, H.H. Jagajīvana Dāsa, H.H. Tamāla Kṛṣṇa Gosvāmī, H.H. Bhagavān Dāsa Mahārāja, and H.H. Kīrtanānanda Swami, among others.

Prabhuji has been honored with various titles and diplomas by many leaders of prestigious religious and spiritual institutions in India. He was given the honorable title *Kṛṣṇa Bhakta* by H.H. Swami Viṣṇu Devānanda (the only title of Bhakti Yoga given by Swami Viṣṇu), disciple of H.H. Swami Śivānanda Sarasvatī and the founder of the Sivananda Organization. He was given the title *Bhaktivedānta* by H.H. B.A. Paramadvaiti Mahārāja, the founder of Vrinda. He was given the title *Yogācārya* by H.H. Swami Viṣṇu Devānanda, the Paramanand Institute of Yoga Sciences and Research of Indore, India, the International Yoga Federation, the Indian Association of Yoga, and the Shri Shankarananda Yogashram of Mysore, India. He received the respectable title *Śrī Śrī Rādhā Śyam Sunder Pāda-Padma Bhakta Śiromaṇi* directly from H.H. Satyanārāyaṇa Dāsa Bābājī Mahant of the Chatu Vaiṣṇava Saṁpradāya.

Prabhuji spent more than forty years studying hatha yoga with prestigious masters in classical and traditional yoga, such as H.H. Bapuji, H.H. Swami Viṣṇu Devānanda Sarasvatī, H.H. Swami Jyotirmayānanda Sarasvatī, H.H. Swami Satchidananda Sarasvatī, H.H. Swami Vignanananda Sarasvatī, and Śrī Madana-mohana.

He attended several systematic hatha yoga teacher training courses at prestigious institutions until he achieved the level of Master Ācārya. He has completed studies at the following institutions: the Sivananda Yoga Vedanta, the Ananda Ashram, the Yoga Research Foundation, the Integral Yoga Academy, the Patanjala Yoga Kendra, the Ma Yoga Shakti International Mission, the Prana Yoga Organization, the Rishikesh Yoga Peeth, the Swami Sivananda Yoga Research Center, and the

Swami Sivananda Yogasana Research Center.

Prabhuji is a member of the Indian Association of Yoga, Yoga Alliance ERYT 500 and YACEP, the International Association of Yoga Therapists, and the International Yoga Federation. In 2014, the International Yoga Federation honored him with the position of Honorary Member of the World Yoga Council.

His interest in the complex anatomy of the human body led him to study chiropractic at the prestigious Institute of Health of the Back and Extremities in Tel Aviv, Israel. In 1993, he received a diploma from Dr. Sheinerman, the founder and director of the institute. Later, he earned a massage therapy diploma at the Academy of Western Galilee. The knowledge he acquired in this field deepened his understanding of hatha yoga and contributed to the creation of his own method.

Retroprogressive Hatha Yoga is the result of Prabhuji's efforts to improve his practice and teaching methods. It is a system based especially on the teachings of his gurus and the sacred scriptures. Prabhuji has systematized various traditional yoga techniques to create a methodology suitable for Western audiences. Retroprogressive Yoga aims to experience our true nature. It promotes balance, health, and flexibility through proper diet, cleansing techniques, preparations (*āyojanas*), sequences (*vinyāsas*), postures (asanas), breathing exercises (*prāṇayama*), relaxation (*śavāsana*), meditation (*dhyāna*), and exercises with locks (*bandhas*) and seals (*mudras*) to direct and empower *prāṇa*.

Since his childhood and throughout his life, Prabhuji

has been an enthusiastic admirer, student, and practitioner of classic karate-do. From the age of 13, he studied different styles in Chile, such as kenpo and kung-fu, but specialized in the most traditional Japanese style of Shotokan. He received the rank of black belt (third dan) from Shihan Kenneth Funakoshi (ninth dan). He also learned from Sensei Takahashi (seventh dan) and practiced Shorin Ryu style with Sensei Enrique Daniel Welcher (seventh dan), who granted him the rank of black belt (second dan). Through karate-do, he delved into Buddhism and gained additional knowledge about the physics of motion. Prabhuji is a member of Funakoshi's Shotokan Karate Association.

Prabhuji grew up in an artistic environment and his love of painting began to develop in his childhood. His father, the renowned Chilean painter Yosef Har-Zion ZT"L, motivated him to devote himself to art. He learned with the famous Chilean painter Marcelo Cuevas. Prabhuji's abstract paintings reflect the depths of the spirit.

Since he was a young boy, Prabhuji has been especially drawn to postal stamps, postcards, mailboxes, postal transportation systems, and all mail-related activities. He has taken every opportunity to visit post offices in different cities and countries. He has delved into the study of philately, the field of collecting, sorting, and studying postage stamps. This passion led him to become a professional philatelist, a stamp distributor authorized by the American Philatelic Society, and a member of the following societies: the Royal Philatelic Society London, the Royal Philatelic Society of Victoria, the United States Stamp Society, the Great Britain Philatelic Society, the American Philatelic Society, the Society of Israel Philatelists, the Society for Hungarian Philately, the National Philatelic Society UK, the Fort Orange Stamp Club, the American Stamp Dealers Association, the US Philatelic Classics Society, FILABRAS – Associação dos Filatelistas Brasileiros, and the Collectors Club of NYC.

Based on his extensive knowledge of philately, theology, and Eastern philosophy, Prabhuji created "Meditative Philately" or "Philatelic Yoga," a spiritual practice that uses philately as the basis for practicing attention, concentration, observation, and meditation. Meditative Philately is inspired by the ancient Hindu *maṇḍala* meditation and it can lead the practitioner to elevated states of consciousness, deep relaxation, and concentration that fosters the recognition of consciousness. Prabhuji wrote his thesis on this new type of yoga, "Meditative Philately," attracting the interest of the Indian academic community due to its innovative way of connecting meditation with different hobbies and activities. For this thesis, he was honored with a PhD in Yogic Philosophy from Yoga-Samskrutum University.

Prabhuji lived in Israel for many years, where he furthered his studies of Judaism. One of his main teachers and sources of inspiration was Rabbi Shalom Dov Lifshitz ZT"L, whom he met in 1997. This great saint guided him for several years on the intricate paths of the Torah and Chassidism. The two developed a very intimate relationship. Prabhuji studied the Talmud with Rabbi Raphael Rapaport Shlit"a (Ponovich), Chassidism with Rabbi Israel Lifshitz Shlit"a, and the Torah with Rabbi Daniel Sandler Shlit"a. Prabhuji is a great devotee of Rabbi Mordechai Eliyahu ZT"L, who personally blessed him.

Prabhuji visited the United States in 2000 and during his stay in New York, he realized that it was the most appropriate place to found a religious organization. He was particularly attracted by the pluralism and respectful attitude of American society toward freedom of religion. He was impressed by the deep respect of both the public and the government for religious minorities. After consulting his master and requesting his blessings, Prabhuji relocated to the United States in 2001. In 2003, the Prabhuji Mission was born, a Hindu church aimed at preserving Prabhuji's universal and pluralistic vision of Hinduism and his Retroprogressive Yoga.

Although he did not seek to attract followers, for 15 years (1995–2010), Prabhuji considered the requests of a few people who approached him asking to become his monastic disciples. Those who chose to see Prabhuji as their spiritual master voluntarily accepted vows of poverty and life-long dedication to spiritual practice (*sadhāna*), religious devotion (*bhakti*), and selfless service (*seva*). Although Prabhuji no longer accepts new disciples, he continues to guide the small group of monastic disciples of the Ramakrishnananda Monastic Order that he founded.

In 2011, Prabhuji founded the Avadhutashram (monastery) in the Catskills Mountains in upstate New York, USA. The Avadhutashram is the headquarters of the Prabhuji Mission, his hermitage, and the residence of the monastic disciples of the Ramakrishnananda Monastic Order. The ashram organizes humanitarian projects such as the Prabhuji Food Distribution Program and the Prabhuji Toy Distribution Program. Prabhuji operates various humanitarian projects, inspired in his experience that serving the part is serving the Whole.

In January 2012, Prabhuji's health forced him to officially renounce managing the mission. Since then, he has lived in solitude, completely away from the public, writing and absorbed in contemplation. He shares his experience and wisdom in books and filmed talks. His message does not promote collective spirituality, but individual inner search.

In 2022, Prabhuji founded the Institute of Retroprogressive Yoga. Here, his most senior disciples can systematically share Prabhuji's teachings and message through video conferences. The institute offers support and help for a deeper understanding of Prabhuji's teachings.

Prabhuji is a respected member of the American Philosophical Association, the American Association of Philosophy Teachers, the American Association of University Professors, the Southwestern Philosophical Society, the Authors Guild, the National Writers Union, PEN America, the International Writers Association, the National Association of Independent Writers and Editors, the National Writers Association, the Alliance Independent Authors, and the Independent Book Publishers Association.

Prabhuji's vast literary contribution includes books in Spanish, English, and Hebrew, for example, *Kundalini Yoga: The Power is in you*, *What is, as it is*, *Bhakti-Yoga: The Path of Love*, *Tantra: Liberation in the World*, *Experimenting with the Truth*, *Advaita Vedanta: Be the Self*, commentaries on the *Īśāvāsya Upanishad* and the *Diamond Sūtra*.

About the Prabhuji Mission

Prabhuji, H.H. Avadhūta Śrī Bhaktivedānta Yogācārya Ramakrishnananda Bābājī Mahārāja, founded the Prabhuji Mission in 2003, a Hindu church aimed at preserving Prabhuji's universal and pluralistic vision of Hinduism.

The main purpose of the mission is to preserve Prabhuji's teachings of Pūrvavyāpi-pragatiśīlaḥ Yoga, or Retroprogressive Yoga, which advocates for a global awakening of consciousness as the radical solution to humanity's problems.

The Prabhuji Mission operates a Hindu temple called Śrī Śrī Radha-Śyāmasundara Mandir, which offers worship and religious ceremonies to parishioners. An extensive library and virtual institute provides religious and spiritual education about many theologies and philosophies for those who want to study Prabhuji's message in depth. The Avadhutashram monastery educates monastic disciples on various aspects of Prabhuji's approach to Hinduism and offers them the opportunity to express devotion to God through devotional service by selflessly contributing their skills and training to the Mission's programs, such as the Prabhuji Food Distribution program, among others.

Service and glorification of the guru are fundamental spiritual principles in Hinduism. The Prabhuji Mission, as a traditional Hindu church, practices the millenary *guru-bhakti* tradition of reverence to the master. Some disciples and friends of the Prabhuji Mission, on their own initiative, help to preserve Prabhuji's legacy and his interfaith teachings for future generations by disseminating his books, videos of his internal talks, and websites

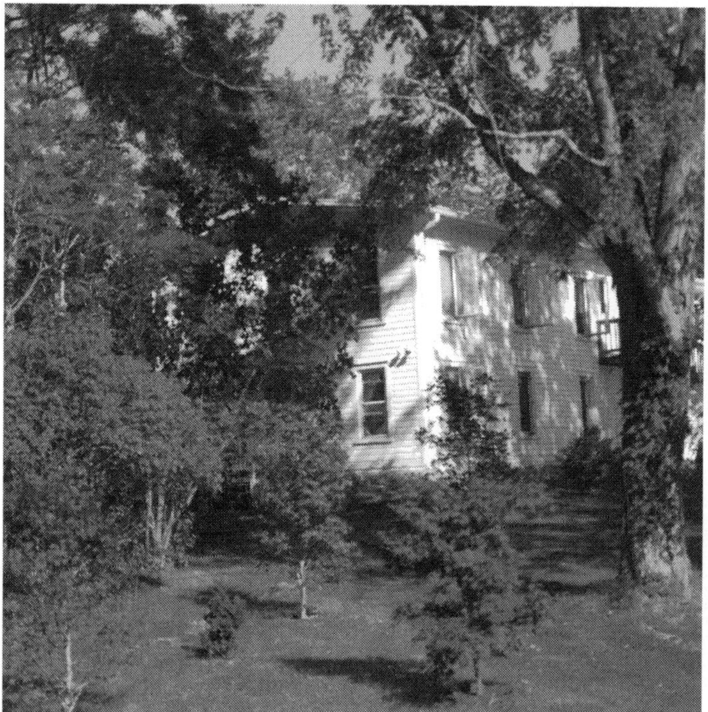

About the Avadhutashram

The Avadhutashram (monastery) was founded by Prabhuji in the Catskills Mountains in upstate New York, USA. It is the headquarters of the Prabhuji Mission and the hermitage of H.H. Avadhūta Śrī Bhaktivedānta Yogācārya Ramakrishnananda Bābājī Mahārāja and his monastic disciples of the Ramakrishnananda Monastic Order.

The ideals of the Avadhutashram are love and selfless service, based on the universal vision that God is in everything and everyone. Its mission is to distribute spiritual books and organize humanitarian projects such as the Prabhuji Food Distribution Program and the Prabhuji Toy Distribution Program.

The Avadhutashram is not commercial and operates without soliciting donations. Its activities are funded by Prabhuji's Gifts, a non-profit company founded by Prabhuji, which sells esoteric items from different traditions that Prabhuji himself has used for spiritual practices during his evolutionary process. Its mission is to preserve and disseminate traditional religious, mystical, and ancestral crafts.

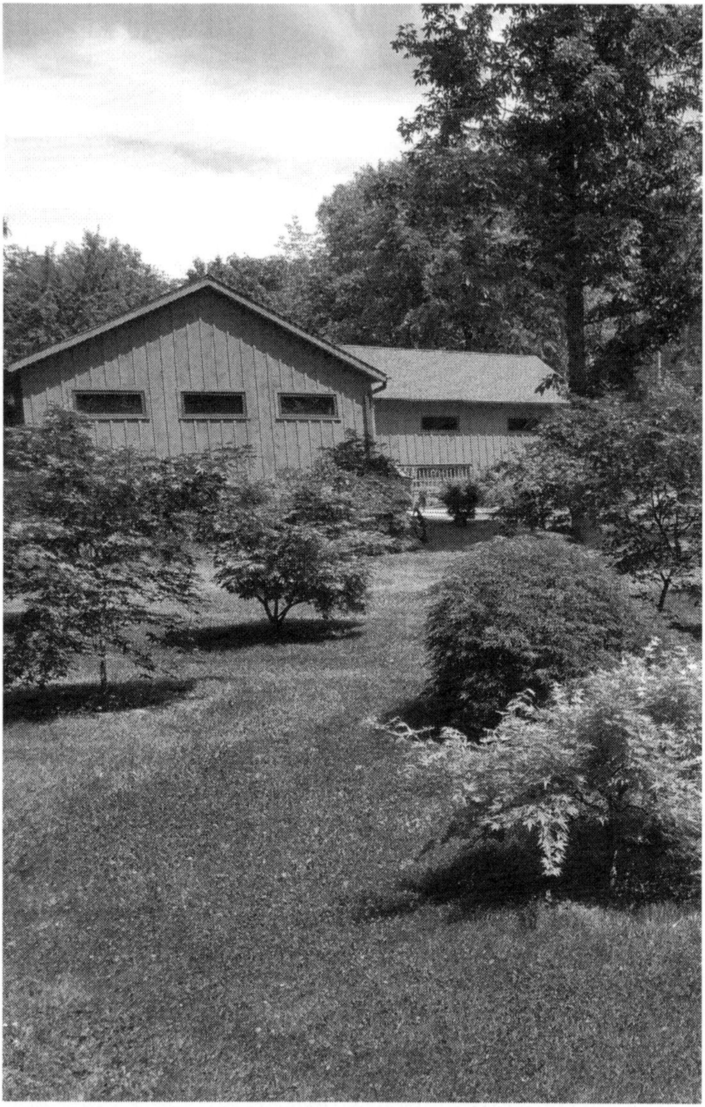

Avadhutashram
Round Top, Nueva York, EE. UU.

The Retroprogressive Path

The Retroprogressive Path does not require you to be part of a group or a member of an organization, institution, society, congregation, club, or exclusive community. Living in a temple, monastery, or *āśram* is not mandatory, because it is not about a change of residence, but of consciousness. It does not urge you to believe, but to doubt. It does not demand you to accept something, but to explore, investigate, examine, inquire, and question everything. It does not suggest being what you should be but being what you really are.

The Retroprogressive Path supports freedom of expression but not proselytizing. This route does not promise answers to our questions but induces us to question our answers. It does not promise to be what we are not or to attain what we have not already achieved. It is a retro-evolutionary path of self-discovery that leads from what we think we are to what we really are. It is not the only way, nor the best, the simplest, or the most direct. It is an involutionary process par excellence that shows what is obvious and undeniable but usually goes unnoticed: that which is simple, innocent, and natural.

It is a path that begins and ends in you.

The Retroprogressive Path is a continuous revelation that expands eternally. It delves into consciousness from a ontologic perspective, transcending all religion and spiritual paths. It is the discovery of diversity as a unique and inclusive reality. It is the encounter of consciousness with itself, aware of itself and its own reality. In fact, this path is a simple invitation to dance in the now, to love the present moment, and to celebrate our authenticity. It is an unconditional proposal to stop living as a victim of circumstance and to live as a passionate adventurer. It is a call to return to the place we have never left, without offering us anything we do not already possess or teaching us anything we do not already know. It is a call for an inner revolution and to enter the fire of life that only consumes dreams, illusions, and fantasies but does not touch what we are. It does not help us reach our desired goal, but instead prepares us for the unexpected miracle.

This path was nurtured over a lifetime dedicated to the search for Truth. It is a grateful offering to existence for what I have received. But remember, do not look for me. Look for yourself. It is not me you need, because you are the only one who really matters. This life is just a wonderful parenthesis in eternity to know and love. What you long for lies in you, here and now, as what you really are.

Your unconditional well-wisher,
Prabhuji

Prabhuji Today

Prabhuji is retired from public life

Prabhuji is the sole disciple of H.D.G. Avadhūta Śrī Brahmānanda Bābājī Mahārāja, who is himself one of the closest and most intimate disciples of H.D.G. Avadhūta Śrī Mastarāma Bābājī Mahārāja.

Prabhuji was appointed as the successor of the lineage by his master, who conferred upon him the responsibility of continuing the line of disciplic succession of *avadhūtas*, or the sacred *paramparā*, officially designating him as guru and commanding him to serve as the successor Ācārya under the name H.H. Avadhūta Śrī Bhaktivedānta Yogācārya Ramakrishnananda Bābājī Mahārāja.

In 2011, he chose to retire from society and lead the life of a hermit. Since then, his days have been spent in solitude, praying, writing, painting, and meditating in silence and contemplation. He no longer participates in *sat-saṅgs*, lectures, gatherings, meetings, retreats, seminars, study groups, or courses. We ask everyone to respect his privacy and do not try to contact him by any means for gatherings, meetings, interviews, blessings, *śaktipāta*, initiations, or personal visits.

Prabhuji's teachings

As a mystic, Hindu *avadhūta*, and realized Spiritual Master, Prabhuji has always appreciated and shared the essence and spiritual wisdom of a wide variety of religious practices from around the world. He does not consider himself a member or representative of any particular religion. Although many see him as an enlightened being, Prabhuji has no intention of presenting himself as a preacher, guide, coach, content creator, influencer, preceptor, mentor, counselor, consultant, monitor, tutor, teacher, instructor, educator, enlightener, pedagogue, evangelist, rabbi, *posek halacha*, healer, therapist, satsangist, psychic, leader, medium, savior, or guru. In fact, Prabhuji believes spirituality is an individual, solitary, personal, private, and intimate search. It is not a collective endeavor to be undertaken through social, organized, institutional, or community religiosity.

To that end, Prabhuji does not proselytize or preach, nor does he try to persuade, convince, or make anyone change their perspective, philosophy, or religion. Instead, he shares his personal view through books and lectures that are available online. Others may find his insights valuable and apply them wholly or in part to their own development, but Prabhuji's teachings are not meant to be seen as personal advice, counseling, guidance, self-help methods, or techniques for spiritual, physical, emotional, or psychological development. He only seeks to share what he has experienced on his own retroprogressive process. His experiences will not provide solutions to life's spiritual, material, financial, psychological, emotional, romantic, family, social, or physical problems. Prabhuji does not promise miracles, mystical experiences, astral journeys, healings, connections with spirits, supernatural powers, or spiritual salvation.

Although he did not seek to attract followers, for 15 years (1995–2010), Prabhuji considered the requests of a few people who approached him asking to become his monastic disciples. Those who chose to see Prabhuji as their spiritual master voluntarily accepted vows of poverty and life-long dedication to spiritual practice (*sādhanā*), religious devotion (*bhakti*), and selfless service (*seva*). Prabhuji no longer accepts new disciples, but he continues to guide the small group of veteran disciples of the Ramakrishnananda Monastic Order that he founded.

Public services

Even though the monastery does not accept new residents, volunteers, donations, collaborations, or sponsorships, the public is cordially invited to participate in daily religious services and attend devotional festivals at the Śrī Śrī Radha-Śyāmasundara Mandir temple.

Titles by Prabhuji

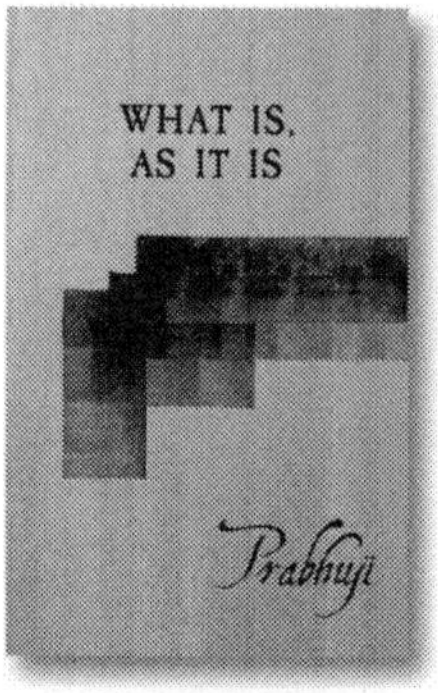

What is, as it is: Satsangs with Prabhuji (English)
ISBN-13:978-0-9815264-4-7
Lo que es, tal como es: Satsangs con Prabhuji (Spanish)
ISBN-13:978-0-9815264-5-4
Russian: ISBN-13: 978-1-945894-18-3

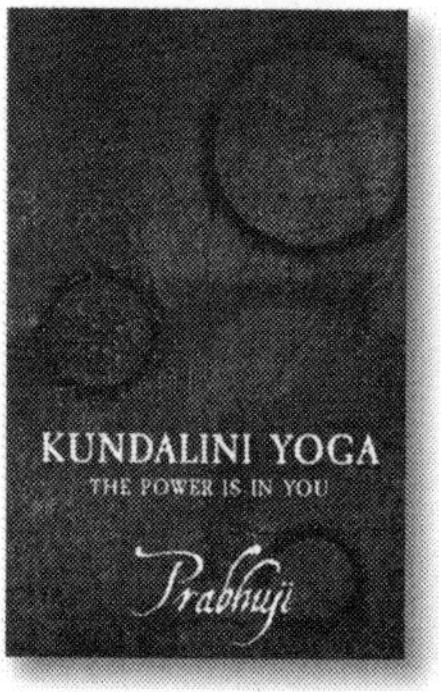

Kundalini yoga: The power is in you (English)
ISBN-13:978-1-945894-02-2
Kundalini yoga: El poder está en ti (Spanish)
ISBN-13:978-1-945894-01-5

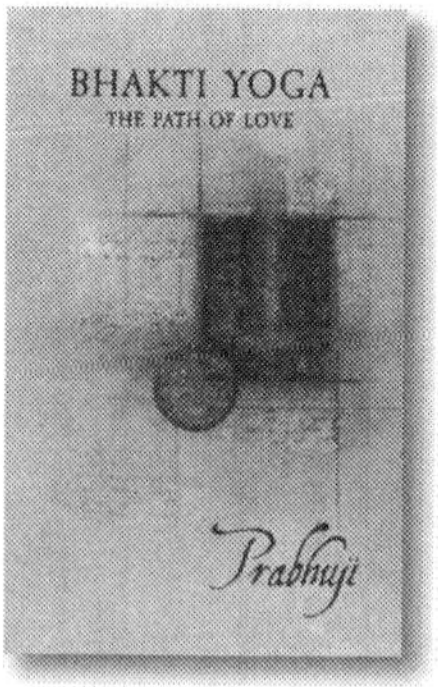

Bhakti yoga: The path of love (English)
ISBN-13:978-1-945894-03-9
Bhakti-yoga: El sendero del amor (Spanish)
ISBN-13:978-1-945894-04-6

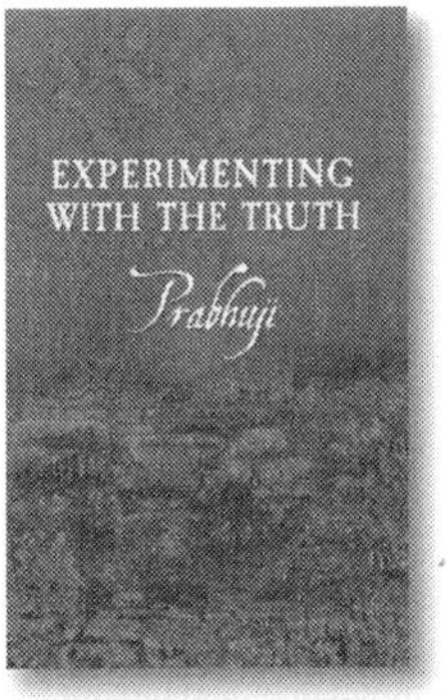

Experimenting with the Truth (English)
ISBN-13: 978-1-945894-08-4
Experimentando con la Verdad (Spanish)
ISBN-13: 978-1-945894-09-1

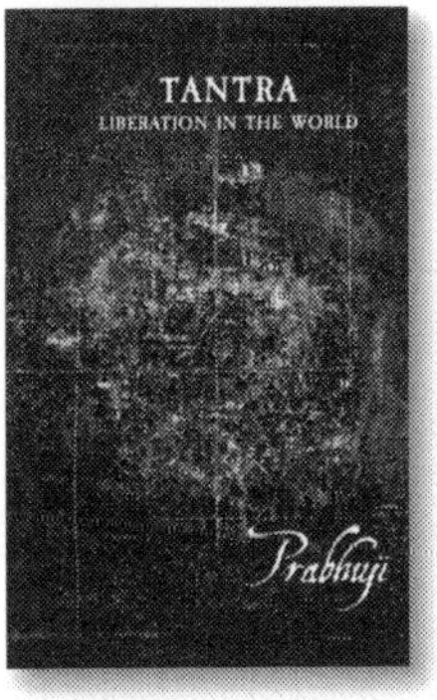

Tantra: Liberation in the world (English)
ISBN-13: 978-1-945894-21-3
Tantra: La liberación en el mundo (Spanish)
ISBN-13: 978-1-945894-23-7

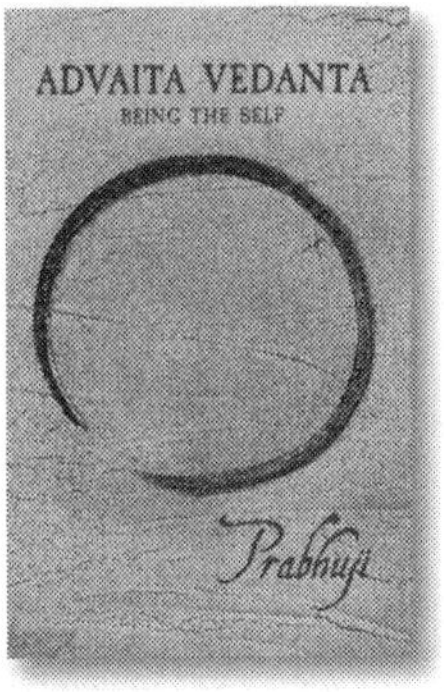

Advaita Vedanta: Being the Self (English)
ISBN-13: 978-1-945894-20-6
Advaita Vedanta: Ser el Ser (Spanish)
ISBN-13: 978-1-945894-16-9

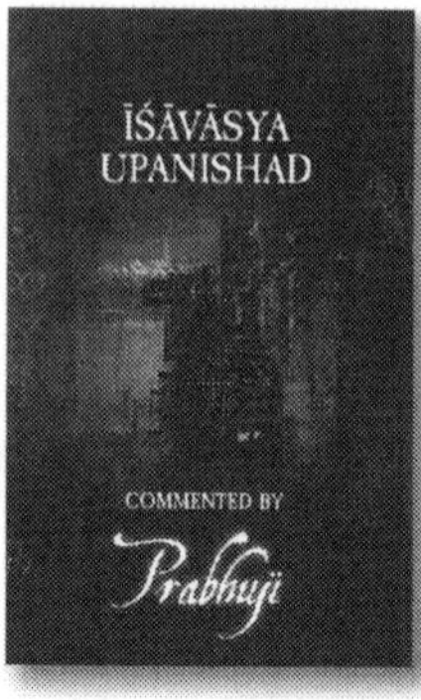

Īśāvāsya Upanishad
commented by Prabhuji
(English)
ISBN-13: 978-1-945894-39-8
Īśāvāsya Upaniṣad
comentado por Prabhuji
(Spanish)
ISBN-13: 978-1-945894-41-1

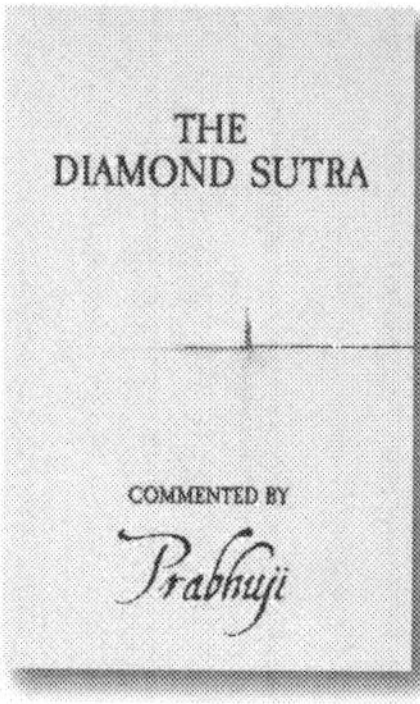

The Diamond Sūtra
commented by Prabhuji
(English)
ISBN-13: 978-1-945894-46-6
El Sūtra del Diamante
comentado por Prabhuji
(Spanish)
ISBN-13: 978-1-945894-49-7

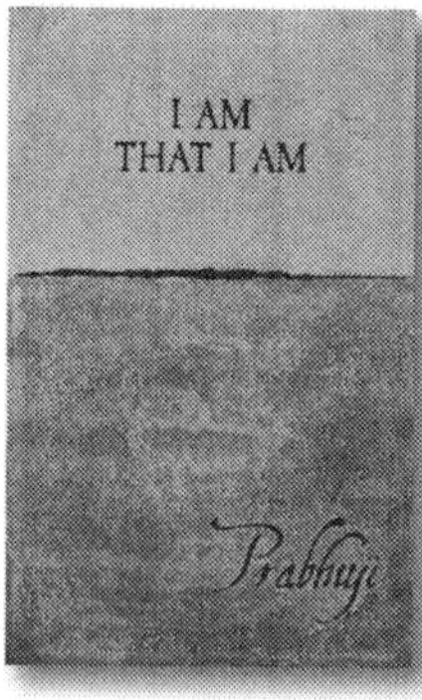

I am that I am
(English)
ISBN-13: 978-1-945894-46-6
Soy el que soy
(Spanish)
ISBN-13: 978-1-945894-49-7

Made in the USA
Middletown, DE
24 February 2023

25268045R00255